Medau

—

THE ART OF ENERGY

Irene F. Chalmers.

The Medau Method is fully supported by the
'Sports Establishment' and Adult Education. The Medau Society
is grant-aided by the Sports Council and is a member of the
Central Council of Physical Recreation.

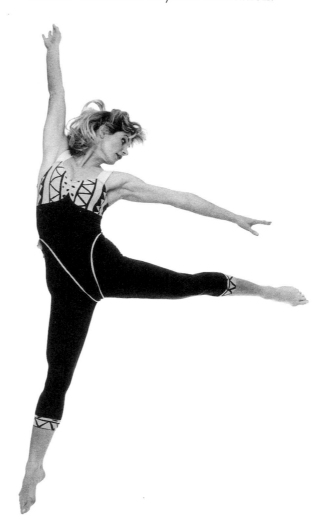

Medau

—
THE ART OF ENERGY

Lucy Jackson

featuring Lala Manners

Thorsons
An Imprint of HarperCollins*Publishers*

Thorsons
An imprint of HarperCollinsPublishers
77-85 Fulham Palace Road
Hammersmith
London W6 8JB

Published by Thorsons 1992

10 9 8 7 6 5 4 3 2 1

A catalogue record for this book
is available from the British Library

ISBN 0 7225 2572 9

Printed in Great Britain by
Butler & Tanner Ltd, Frome, Somerset

Contents

Foreword: Dame Ninette de Valois   9

Preface: Dr Jochen Medau   11

1   Medau: What is it?   13

2   The Magic of Medau: A Personal Discovery   15

3   The Changing Face of Medau   20

4   The Health Benefits of Medau   29

5   The Way a Class Works   43

The Art of Energy

6   Using the Art of Energy   51

7   Warm Up   56

8   Stretch: the Energy of Water   61

9   Strength: the Energy of Earth   71

10   Stamina: the Energy of Fire   79

11   Suppleness: the Energy of Air   85

12   Wind Down   96

Adapting Medau

13   Medau for the Under 5s   103

14   Medau for the Over 40s   108

15   Medau for the Over 60s   110

16   Medau Through Your Pregnancy   112

17   Whole Body Harmony   117

    Professional Tributes   119

Acknowledgements

My special thanks to my daughter Lala Manners for her collaboration with the text and for producing the beautiful pictures for this book.

Thanks to Claire Griffiths and Joanna Gibbon for their help with the manuscript.

Thanks to 'my teachers' – the remarkable women who taught me, especially Molly Braithwaite, Hildegard Erbguth, Hella Thommen and Jutta Holler von der Trenk.

To my Medau friends and fellow teachers.

To my friends and colleagues in the Laban Guild.

To the Medau family for their friendship and encouragement over many years.

For Senta

Foreword

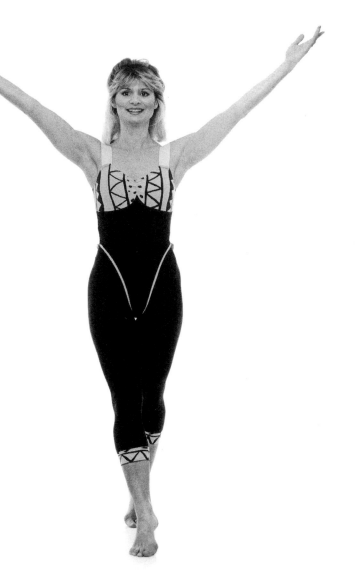

The work of the Medau Society should most certainly be placed alongside the other famous health, beauty and exercise groups that have sprung from the contemporary dance movement all over Europe.

I found the videotape of this particular method very fascinating and enjoyable and so well executed by Lala Manners. The book will be of interest to all of us who take the execution of modern dance and natural movement seriously. I wish it and the Medau Society every success.

Dame Ninette de Valois CH.DBE
Patron of the Medau Society

Preface

—

Dr Jochen Medau is the younger son of Hinrich and Senta Medau.
He is Principal of the Medau College and a practising consultant cardiologist.

I am delighted to have been asked to write the Preface for this lovely book.

It provides an excellent and authentic account of my parents' work in the past and a real vision of its importance and application in the future.

Lucy's knowledge and enthusiasm shines through every page and my father's ever-questing spirit would have relished her passion for finding new ways to develop his work. She proves the truth of his saying 'My future existence lies in the hands of my teachers.' Building on Molly Braithwaite's work in Britain, Lucy has opened up a whole new world for Medau. Her legendary skill as a teacher and her ability to inspire others, give her work a special significance. The length of her active teaching career and the extraordinary range and scope of her experience, make her one of our most versatile and widely travelled 'ambassadors'.

She has in her daughter, Lala, a brilliant colleague and exponent of the Medau technique. I am lost in admiration of her beauty and skill in the video film *Medau: the Art of Energy* and in the photography of this book.

This combined project of video and book is a major step in bringing my father's work to a much wider public. It retains all the hallmarks of his original concept, but is presented in a style which is completely contemporary and accessible to all.

I am always deeply touched by Lucy's love and loyalty to my parents. I can truly say that, from the time that I remember her as a student at the school, the admiration and affection was always mutual.

We send both Lucy and Lala our

formal congratulations and best
wishes from the College. From my
wife, Ingrid, my sister Katerina and
from myself, we send our thanks
and greetings of love and
friendship.

Jochen Medau, Coburg
January 1991

1 *Medau: What is it?*

Medau —

What is it?

Imagine a panther . . .

*and try to describe it. The words you use
will fit the description of all that Medau
seeks to achieve.*

A strong, lithe body
perfectly designed for action
moving effortlessly
full of ease and elegance
powerful but unstressed
harmonious and balanced in
mind and body
true to itself
efficient, economical and built to last.

Are you smiling?

Hinrich Medau turned to the strength and grace of animals for inspiration on how the body ought to move.

He believed that movement which is natural and right for the body will look easy.

The first aim of Medau is to teach the body to move 'correctly'. Maximum efficiency should be achieved with the least amount of effort. There should be no distortion or jolting, but a strong

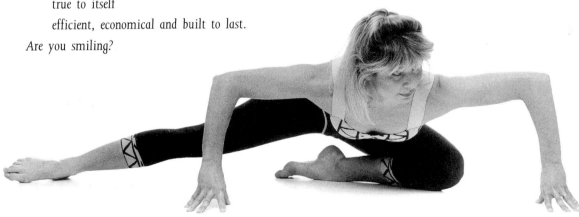

flow of rhythm through the whole body to achieve the ultimate in fluid coordination.

The Art of Energy is an effective, safe and fun programme expertly structured to develop stretch, strength, stamina and suppleness. In following it you will discover your own natural ease, energy, rhythm and enjoy the total involvement of mind and body.

Medau works *with* the body, not against it. All the movements are simple and 'natural' to the body, so that anyone can have a go!

Boost your vitality, feel confident and enjoy the full potential of your life.

Medau is for you.

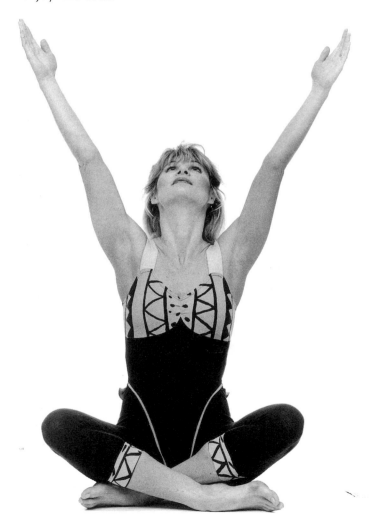

2 *The Magic of Medau*

A PERSONAL DISCOVERY

It is astonishing to think that Medau was for me a chance meeting which, though unplanned and seemingly unimportant at the time, has shaped and influenced my life for almost forty years.

I was in my early twenties. Just out of university, where tennis and other activities had satisfied my modest need for exercise, I was looking for a new winter pastime. Scottish reels had always been fun and I looked for an evening class. With the usual muddle-making of youth, I discovered the local Adult Education Institute on the wrong night, and was persuaded to try the new movement class instead. I was not pleased, protesting that my dancing skirt was too long, my knickerbockers too tight, and any-way, what *was* this movement class?

Though naturally energetic I was no great athlete, and a very indifferent games player. I was certainly not about to join a fitness or exercise programme, and viewed it with some suspicion.

The teacher was small and neat. Dressed in a sky blue tunic, she seemed to achieve an extraordinary feat of virtuosity, demonstrating large, simple swinging movements to the class, then sprinting to a handy piano which she played with some skill.

This was something genuinely different. There were no piano renderings from the shows, no repeated mechanical 'trim the waist' bends so popular at that time. There was nothing to offend or stir my heightened sense of the ridiculous. This ordinary group of people in an ordinary school hall seemed filled with ease and elegance. What was this strange compelling rhythm which urged me to run, spring and stretch with such curious pleasure?

It stirred a scene from my childhood. I remembered that once, as a small girl, I had skipped out across the grass with the Maypole dancers. Too tiny to manage the ribbons, we little ones were meant to retire quietly and watch the dancing. Filled with enthusiasm, I failed to stop, and danced on, completely absorbed, spreading heedless chaos amongst the flying ribbons. When finally removed and carried off aloft, I seemed not to notice, and went on skipping in the air, finishing only to weep with disappointment when the music stopped.

Something of that excitement and strange elemental compulsion to move with the rhythm struck me again in that first Medau class. This response has remained as a source of pleasure and wonder ever since.

The teacher of that first class was the great Molly Braithwaite, who made it her life work to establish the Medau Method in Britain. It was she who suggested I should do a summer course, followed by a year's study at the Medau School in Coburg, Germany. Founded by Hinrich and Senta Medau in 1929, the school was renowned for its advanced ideas about health, fitness

and teacher training for women. At the very heart of their thinking was the importance of music and rhythmical movement.

It is difficult to exaggerate the impact Hinrich and Senta Medau had on me. With the memory of lumpy games teachers fresh in my mind, I marvelled that these people could be so glorious and glamorous. Musical, cultured, handsome and charming, they ruled the school with an astonishing mix of warm affection and absolute authority. Dazzled by the Medau magic, I was absorbed into a way of life very alien to my reserved and gently cynical English self.

I was astonished to discover that personal health concerns were openly discussed and considered important. Until then my only concession to a health regime had been a daily shot of fresh air and an apple. I was not *sure* of my sleep patterns, energy levels and special dietary needs, let alone the best way to trim my toe nails or scrub my knees and elbows with a string glove! Everything 'mattered' to the Medaus who seemed to cultivate a sensitivity and awareness about life which altered fundamentally my rather brisk and British matter-offactness.

'Rhythmic Movement' was only one part, albeit essential, of the wide syllabus. Athletics, volleyball and even conducting the choir had to be tackled and mastered. In time I developed a greater level of rhythmic coordination and general fitness through the movement training, so that I could attempt even vaulting and somersaults which had terrified me in my own school days in the gym.

Returning to London the following summer, I knew that with the Medaus one of the great links of my life had been forged. From that time until now, I have taught continuously and kept in close contact with the school in Coburg. Like all their students, I adored the Medaus, and even now, twenty years after Senta's death, I feel the influence of her affection and draw upon the brilliance of her inspired teaching.

I studied in London for the British Medau Diploma with my original teacher, Molly Braithwaite, who had been trained by the Medaus before World War II. She had used the 'rhythmic movement' part of their work to create 'recreational classes', as they were then called.

Educated at a Quaker school, and then at Newnham College, Cambridge, Molly had a highly developed dedication to the social good. She taught us the craft of teaching, inspiring us with her own missionary zeal. Our enthusiasm was unshakeable. We had a shining purpose, a message which neither small groups and winter snows nor summer heat could dim.

It was a happy time for me. Recently married, I had time to explore other movement theories. I learned dance with Ernst and Lotte Birk and the Laban Dance method with Christa Haring. There were large set piece displays at Wembley and the Royal Albert Hall, and lecture demonstrations up and down the country. I learnt through Molly's example to teach anyone, anywhere. No circumstance was too difficult and no opportunity too inconvenient. Teaching all over the world, as I do now, when the going gets tough and 'planes are late or time zones zap my energy, I think of Molly and remember the tenacity, stamina and courage of a remarkable woman.

My daughter Lala was born in 1960, and twin sons, Julian and

James, in 1962. I do love, and have always loved, the whole business of childhood. Even considering the inevitable anxieties and frequent exhaustion, it is still an enchanted time. Music, movement and dance were an on-going festival and my children's nursery 'class' at home with Lala and her brothers was a daily affair – not that we set it up as such, but there is no doubt in my mind that the work that Lala and I have subsequently created for children derives in large part from these childhood years (see page 103).

I took Lala to the Medau School when she was five. There she pottered and played, joining in sometimes or sitting on top of the grand piano in the enormous gym. She remembers the Medaus at this time, especially Senta and her warm and lovely smile.

There were early signs of a passion for movement and Lala's first school report still makes me laugh. 'Lanya Mary has a beautifully compact and balanced body, well suited to dance. Her enthusiasm and enviable sense of rhythm make her a joy to teach. She must, however, learn to move with the group, as her talent for improvisation tends to confuse the other dancers. A+', signed Tessie Hutchinson. I was reminded of another small girl dancing with absorbed delight amongst the Maypole ribbons.

At school she grew more interested in games, but returned to dance before university, when she studied with Ernst Birk and his second wife, Ailsa, specialists in dance and percussion. After her degree Lala taught in primary schools for a while, but soon discovered that her real joy was teaching the children movement rather than the three Rs and so quickly changed direction.

Medau has been an authentic and continuous influence throughout Lala's life so it was no surprise that she made this decision. As a supremely gifted and joyful mover, her rare combination of artistry and athleticism is typical of the original Medau concept. With the advantage of never having had to unlearn anything her development has been easy and organic. She has emerged as a top teacher and presenter of the work. A skilled and successful grass roots teacher with a wide range of experience, it is these qualities which will guide you easily through the Medau programme whether you follow it here or on the video.

Lala's small daughter Harriet, with a child's delight in her own energy and increasing physical competence, reminds me constantly

that it is not only for fitness and trim figures that Medau is famous. After the last expert word has been said about pulse rates and cellulite, loading the joints and stretching the muscles, movement is about the instinctive development of the whole person, an on-going adventure of increased ease, self-confidence and pleasure.

When asked 'Why Medau?', I reply, 'Because it makes people happy.' That, in the end, is the best reason I have ever known.

3   *The Changing Face of Medau*

How it all began

It seems impossible to fully enjoy the Art of Energy without developing an interest in the background to Medau's work. What were the influences which shaped this astonishing man? How did the Medau School develop?

Hinrich Medau always said that the true origins of his work lay in his childhood on a farm – in Schleswig-Holstein, the most northern part of Germany. He and his friends, with all the exuberance of youth, moved freely through the countryside practising natural gymnastics in the way of all young creatures.

Always strong and immensely energetic, with an outstanding musical talent, he trained to become a music and gymnastic teacher, and later travelled to Portugal in order to gain some teaching experience. There the grace and ease of movement of the Portuguese people were to make a lasting impression on him. In the early 1920s when the new, freer, whole body movement was being taught and talked about in Germany and Scandinavia, it struck an immediate chord of recognition. Medau was full of enthusiasm for the new ideas in education – particularly the 'new look' rhythmical movement for women, which was beginning to supercede 'free-standing' exercise in the more enterprising physical education colleges.

He retrained and studied these new ideas at the Bode school which pioneered some of the first work on free movement. There he met and married a fellow student. Senta was a remarkable woman and her influence on his work was to be immense. They left with a small band of brilliantly gifted teachers to found their own school in Berlin in 1929. Every new idea in dance, sport and music came under Medau's scrutiny. And very soon the Medau School became famous for its free-thinking and advanced ideas on health, fitness and teacher training.

Although his work was firmly rooted in physical education, there were new developments in four other main areas which also had a major influence on the evolution of his ideas. Innovative figures in the fields of general education, music, dance and theatre were to be an inspiration to Hinrich.

Zeitgeist!

To understand how this 'new movement' had arrived, we need to consider the Zeitgeist, or Spirit of the Time, at the turn of this century. With industrialization and the growth of cities throughout Europe, more and more people left the countryside to live in cramped houses in crowded back streets. Working long hours in mills, mines and factories, it seemed that people were losing their contact with the earth – with their roots, if you like – and the cry of 'Back to Nature' went up.

This new attitude was reflected in all aspects of life:

The development of Art Nouveau, with its swirling, organic forms, symbolized growth and the natural rhythms of wind and water.

There was a revival of interest in handcraft, folk music and dance, because it was felt that people denied the traditional ways of expressing their creativity would lose something of their essential human nature. Spontaneity, enthusiasm, being in touch with nature, self-expression and openness to life became the fashion, a far cry from the more stilted, rigid work based on 19th-century mores.

In the field of education, teachers began to question the effect of the strict, punishment-based rigours of the Victorian schoolroom. Was there not a more 'natural' way to stimulate and teach young bodies and minds? Froebel, Steiner and Maria Montessori were but a few of the great pioneers who insisted on 'freeing the child' to develop at his or her own pace without toil or fear.

Meanwhile, in the world of dance, Isadora Duncan had cast off her shoes (and her corsets!) and in whirling chiffon and with passionate emotion had convinced her audiences that nature, truth and art were one. She danced to 'the rhythms of nature' responding to the elements of earth, fire, water and air. Her impact on the world of dance was immense, and there is little doubt that these frissons of delight were felt throughout the world of physical education too. The rigid, mechanical, repetitive exercises looked suddenly archaic and dead. The concept of flowing, rhythmical movement for women was born.

The Development of Medau Movement

Imagine the effect on Hinrich Medau at this time – a brilliant young man searching for new ideas. It was not enough to say that these ideas looked right, felt right and expressed contemporary attitudes. How on earth did one achieve them? Isadora simply danced, and even her work with children (known as the Isadorables) owed more to inspiration than formal teaching method.

The new cinematograph (the early cine camera) provided him with one clue. The movement of dancers, athletes and animals could now be studied on film. This was how the Medaus came up with some basic descriptive terms for the sort of movement they were trying to achieve. They discovered that natural movement has a continuous flow of preparation for the strong impulse or thrust of a movement, followed by recovery or outflow. It seemed like a continuous wave, rising and falling towards gravity and away, with a free floating turning point where the whole body seemed almost weightless. They used words like 'dynamic', 'continuous', 'elastic' and 'resilient', 'economical', 'organic' (that is, arising from deep within the body structure), 'unstressed' and 'involving the whole body as one piece'. It is quite amazing to think that this description of correct movement still holds good today.

Medau had shown a prodigious musical talent from early childhood. 'Instant music' was unknown in those days, and he used to tell us how, as a boy, he would dash home after following the local brass band around, and entertain his family by playing variations of their music on the piano he had begged his father to buy for him.

As a music student, Jacques Dalcroze had shown him that his students' sense of musical rhythm was greatly enhanced when they were taught how to move and to express the rhythm with their bodies. He had devised a system which he called Eurythmics, which also included a method of piano improvization, based on the basic chord patterns of European music.

Medau, by a brilliant leap of creative thinking, adapted this concept and taught his gymnastic students to move more freely through training their response to rhythm. The much-praised flexible and creative use of music and rhythm in fitness classes today owes a lot to

Hinrich Medau's early inspiration.

Medau became very impressed by the dancer Rudolph Laban's work on the analysis of human movement. Laban's themes of shape, space and dynamics in movement, together with his brilliant analysis of the rules of choreography, were profoundly influential on the way Medau presented his work.

Important also was the work of the French theatre producer François Delsarte. Delsarte had found that by teaching his company to swing Indian clubs in large pendulum-like movements, rather than continuing with the jerky army exercises so entrenched at the time, they seemed to move more naturally on stage.

It is this heritage which has provided a richness and variety in Medau's work, making it brilliant and varied in all spheres of movement and dance today. The combination of influences led him, with his team of teachers, to pioneer new and exciting ways to teach movement – using hand apparatus.

The idea of using balls, hoops and clubs made use of every school's basic equipment, and the special method of using hand apparatus to aid good movement was set in motion. Expertly imaginative presentation of large choreographed set-piece displays at international events soon brought him renown as a teacher, and his school to the forefront of physical education in Germany.

Hinrich Medau was a born free thinker and innovator. The concept of his work changing and evolving to suit the special needs of the time was crucial to his thinking and echoed in his constant plea to his students to 'develop my work or I will become a museum piece'. His success is reflected in the great variety and scope of Medau teachers' work today.

The basic principles of Medau Movement as strong, dynamic, rhythmic and involving the whole body have remained absolute. It is the presentation and application only which change, chameleon-like, to suit each special circumstance.

His work has crossed the range from contemporary dance to remedial therapy – from the famous Jutta Czundas Dance Company in Nuremburg, to the highly valued work for the Back Pain Association in England. Certainly I have seen many changes in its scope and application since I began teaching in the 1950s.

The Changing Face of Medau

Whenever I see films or photographs of Medau's work in the early 1930s, I am immediately struck by how absolutely right it looks for the time. The work is light and springy, with the students so pretty in short, soft tunics, bare legs and bobbed hair. The music is melodic and rhythmical, somewhere between the divinity of Schubert and the popularity of the foxtrot. It may seem quaint and dated now, but if we compare it with anything achieved in gymnastics for women before that time we realize how utterly different and completely modern this easy swinging movement must have seemed.

After the despair of World War II, the Medaus, with enormous courage and faith in their work, reopened the school in Flensburg, not far from where Medau was born. These were desperate years,

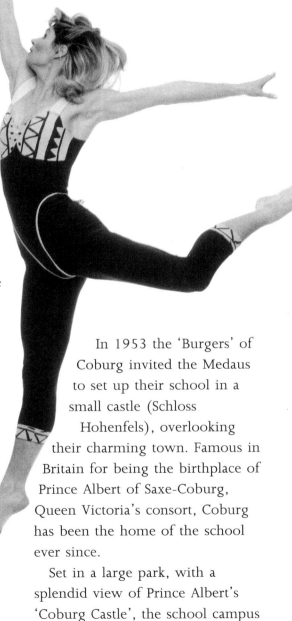

with a young family to bring up and the whole country in a state of confusion, struggling to recover from the war. Looking now at pictures of his students taken on the Flensburg beaches, I marvel at their sparkling vitality even in such difficult days.

This was the time when I went to the school, the movement was larger and grander, and more athletic. Women were competing at international level in sport and athletics, more women had full- or part-time jobs and were playing a more assertive, versatile role outside the home. In any case, the German schools' curriculum was geared to sport and athletics.

The work with hand apparatus was paramount and much of the movement was done in full extension. They performed large swinging movements, running and leaping with speed and strength that would have dazzled the flappers of the 1920s and 1930s.

I have ecstatic memories of flying round the gym hurling hoops into the air and scooping them up again, driven on by the intoxicating piano playing of Medau himself.

In 1953 the 'Burgers' of Coburg invited the Medaus to set up their school in a small castle (Schloss Hohenfels), overlooking their charming town. Famous in Britain for being the birthplace of Prince Albert of Saxe-Coburg, Queen Victoria's consort, Coburg has been the home of the school ever since.

Set in a large park, with a splendid view of Prince Albert's 'Coburg Castle', the school campus is idyllic with gardens, woods and fields of wild flowers. The original

Schloss remains and there are many new buildings for student accommodation, lecture theatres, physiotherapy rooms, gyms and a swimming pool. It is a buzzing, busy student community.

In line with the concept that good movement must, by definition, be correct for the body (see page 22), the school now offers a course which combines movement and training in physiotherapy. This is a unique and influential course which, true to the Medau tradition, has broken new ground and attracts much interest and many 'expert' visitors from all over the world.

The kindness and hospitality of the Familie Medau and their staff, and the continuing standards of excellence set by Hinrich and Senta, still make each visit to the school in Coburg an unforgettable and life-enhancing experience.

There was a major change of emphasis in the 1960s, when young people's self-image was different. Flower Power, meditation and breathing therapy were in vogue, together with introspection and visits to sit at the feet of gurus. Pacifism and the new notion of 'caring' made for a more passive approach.

Senta Medau pulled the work into line with these new trends by placing the emphasis on the breathing and stretch techniques based on yoga positions. Ideas of inner movement, group rhythms, relating to partners, relaxation and inner energy were popular. This work has had a lasting effect on the way we look at movement today, and is very much reflected in the final piece of the Art of Energy, where the strong, smooth, organic movement calms and harmonizes mind and body.

I remember teaching at this time with my hair teased up into a beehive or over my shoulders in immaculate flick-ups. I would finish class with every lacquered strand in place. Sweat and dishevelment would have been unacceptable, just as an hour's worth of softly spoken suggestions from the teacher to 'feel the breathing in your thighs' would seem laughable today.

With the 1970s came the dance craze, glitzy gear and clever routines. Classes required more pace and drama; disco music and high stamina routines dealt the final blow to Flower Power.

Jane Fonda's workouts heralded the much abused and misused 'aerobic exercise' of the early 1980s. There was nothing new in the content of aerobics classes. Running and springing had always been part of our work, but the quantity, intensity and extraordinary noise, and the cheer leader teachers seemed to reflect the aggression and assertiveness of the peak of the women's movement. Their mixed classes, sweat and screams were bound to affect us, and it was at this stage that I reluctantly stopped using the piano in any of the classes. I replaced it with taped music, increased the pace and held on.

The style became stronger and heavier in the late 1980s, with the influence of gym workouts and hand weights, and the dreaded body sculpting. Tightening, toning and the problem areas of buttocks, thighs and abdomen receive special treatment in a way that would have been unthinkable when I started teaching, and anathema to the waif-like Twiggies of the 1960s.

The aerobics craze has now levelled out and the importance of safe fitness linked to proper scientific studies of how the body actually achieves a better performance has become the new angle.

More in line with athletics training and Medau's original teaching, I have been very interested to present a valid fitness class based on movement. Gone are the days of two-hour classes punctuated with tea and chat! People now are looking for an hour's 'fitness package' which is safe and effective. This adaptation has proved one of the most successful. It is an effective blend of the fitness factors (see page 29), plus the elements of correct movement. I have presented this type of class literally all over the world to teachers of dance, exercise and various physical therapies, with great popular success.

Where do we go from here? Well, I'm not quite sure, except that I know we will get it spot on right.

Certainly, Medau is still as relevant in the dance studios or the school hall as it is in the home, taught by video. 'Do-it-yourself fitness' is a vast new area which Medau teachers are exploring with the same integrity of principle and flair for catching the look and specific needs of the time.

Nothing is lost. With each new decade the work evolves and I look forward to a time when natural whole body movement not only contributes as it does today, but provides the basis and the starting point for all dance, fitness and exercise training courses. It makes good sense – training the body is as much a matter of intuition and art as it is of science. Basic movement patterns are learned instinctively and this is where we all begin.

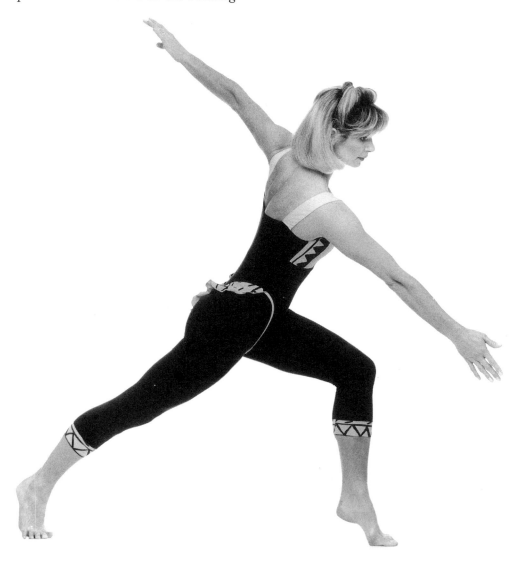

4 *The Health Benefits of Medau*

Remember the Panther

The strength and grace of animals were Hinrich Medau's inspiration on how the body should move, and the first aim of Medau is to teach the body to move correctly.

By developing natural ease, energy and rhythm, and working towards total involvement of the mind and body, you will learn movement which is natural and right for your body. Once achieved, it looks easy, demonstrating maximum efficiency with the least amount of effort.

The Art of Energy is based around four fitness factors – Stretch, Strength, Stamina and Suppleness – which, although different in emphasis and style, all aim to work your body as a whole. It is an effective, safe and fun programme expertly structured to work with your body, not against it.

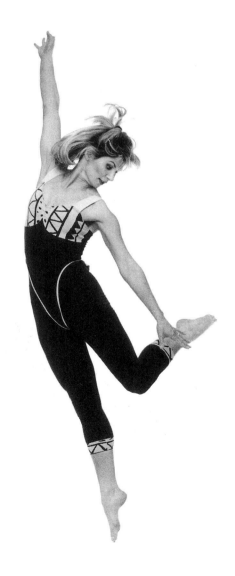

All the movements are simple and natural to the body so that anyone, at whatever level of fitness, can use the programme. As you improve you will respond more intensely to the rhythm of the music which allows you a feeling of greater control and freedom: at this stage you will see and feel the benefits of an improved, firmer body shape. Once you feel this confidence and harmony, the sky is the limit and the programme can be done with ever-increasing effort and effectiveness.

You will find the subtle changes of rhythm, shape and intensity of the movements promote a flow of energy and a deep sense of enjoyment. This programme is not about gritting your teeth and performing like a machine. You should start at your own level, give yourself time to grow into the programme and have realistic long- and short-term goals.

What are the Benefits?

The Ideal Shape

Fashions in body shape come and go. Compare the frail Twiggie look of the 1960s with the solid sweating funkers of the 1980s. Now in the 1990s it seems that a sleaker, more streamlined shape is in demand: the rock hard, often lumpy, muscles of the 1980s need to be toned down. The Medau body is lean, lithe and cat-like; a strong, seamless body-stocking with no over-developed muscles.

Weight distribution and muscle tension should be as even as possible throughout the body, placing no extra stress on bones and joints. The result should be a practical, easy, natural, working body which looks good in every situation.

Remember, you cannot change the bone structure of your body. Body type is largely genetic and it is important to personal well-being to learn to enjoy your body the way it is. However, a strong body which is not carrying excess weight is a key to good health and you can discover your ideal body shape by toning your muscles and diminishing body fat.

This programme will encourage your muscles to strengthen and to develop into a smooth and elongated shape. Each set of muscles affects a specific part of your body: for instance, the strong elastic girdle of the back and abdominal muscles will keep the waist slim and the abdomen flat. Because muscles are inter-related, imbalances can occur if one set becomes over-developed at the expense of others. The Art of Energy ensures that all muscles are worked in harmony.

A certain amount of underlying fat is natural to the female shape, although distribution and amounts do vary from person to person. Some body fat can be reduced during aerobic exercise if it is done regularly and sustained for at least twenty minutes at a time. If weight loss is a major concern, the stamina section should be practised often and, of course, it helps to reduce your calorie intake too.

By maintaining the heart rate, effort and muscle tone in every movement as you exercise, your body will begin gradually to burn up some fat. Soft bulges will trim down and your body will be freed from carrying unwanted extra weight which can stress joints.

As you maintain your exercise programme your bottom, thighs, abdomen and upper arms will begin to shape up and slim down. The end result will be a more defined, firmer look to your figure from tighter muscles and reduced underlying fat.

Maximum Energy

In Medau, personal energy is the starting point for exercise. A streamlined body in tune with itself will waste no energy. Every movement you make will grow naturally from your body wasting no energy. Your body will work in harmony to maximum effect while not being harmfully over-taxed. Think of a perfect shot with a tennis racket which sends the ball soaring over the net.

Understanding this concept of Medau is not complicated but it does involve your getting to know your own body rhythm. As you progress with the Art of Energy you will begin to feel the difference between doing movements that feel right and those that feel uncomfort-able. Discovering the pace which feels right for you will make all tasks easier, and you will discover how to make beneficial changes to your everyday movements as well.

Maximum energy is an essential part of all four workouts, but the Stamina section demonstrates its effect most clearly. Here, maximum effort and maximum ease work together by using your body's natural spring: the result is more energy to continue the programme and a wonderful feeling of lightness and alertness at the end.

The energy of movement can be seen in terms of the four elements:

Earth energy = strength – for weight-bearing and endurance. It involves mainly the large muscle groups such as the back, abdominals, buttocks and thighs. It is the centre of gravity through which you feel the pull and strength of the earth and it makes you feel confident, strong, rooted and able to stand your ground.

Water energy = stretch. It implies the strong, continuous currents which flow through the mind and body, uniting, harmonizing, avoiding stress and

wasted effort. It involves keeping the joints supple, the muscles stretched and the body moving freely. It makes you adaptable, flexible and able to survive.

Fire energy = stamina. It represents heat and high aerobic energy. It involves increasing the heart rate, stimulating the body to a pitch of excitement through stepping, springing, dancing and running. It increases your driving power to achieve new skills, realize ambitions and live with passion and panache.

Air energy = suppleness, calm and inner strength. It involves breathing deeply using the air to sustain and lighten your body, releasing you from the pressure of gravity. It refreshes, revitalizes your mind and develops your sense of spiritual awareness.

A Versatile Body

Modern living demands high levels of skill and fitness. Our lives are complex. We are preoccupied with work, home, relationships – where we juggle various roles, attempting not to be too exhausted at the end of each day. Whether you have a demanding career, a young baby, a time-consuming sport or interest, the need for a reliable, versatile working body is essential so that you can tackle all of life's challenges.

Tailoring fitness to your needs is vital to the success of any exercise programme. Most people want sufficient basic health and fitness to maintain their life, cope with stress and emergencies, and to have enough in reserve for some sort of personal growth. Others want to combine all of the above with more specific aims.

Decide first of all what you need from your fitness programme. Are you about to go on a strenuous skiing or walking holiday? Have you just started a new sport or dance class? Or are you always out of breath when you run for the bus or climb the stairs?

This programme produces a sound, strong body which will be prepared to try anything or can enhance a present activity. The strength and agility you achieve with the Art of Energy will directly aid general sports and athletics as well as holiday pastimes, such as windsurfing and skiing.

A fit, correctly aligned body is less prone to injury. General flexibility makes life's tasks easier,

from carrying small children, coping with the rough and tumble of their games, painting and decorating and even housecleaning.

And lastly, basic fitness heightens your sense of well-being, making you mentally stronger and able to cope with life's challenges. For example, a strong body will help during pregnancy, birth and post-natal recovery (see Pregnancy, page 112).

Stress Control

Medau has been described as meditation in movement. It teaches you to relax. The unstressed body makes for an unstressed mind and the strong, dynamic, rhythmical movements of Medau will gradually bring you calmness and confidence.

You will discover that this is not a conscious process. As you move and concentrate on different parts of your body you will get to know yourself and gradually you will unwind. The combination of music and harmonious and rhythmic movements will take your mind away from the worries and strains of life: tensions will disappear as muscles warm, stretch and relax.

You will find that your mind switches off from your problems –

which will benefit both mind and body. A particularly high-pressure situation, with no let up, does not simply cause mental stress but will manifest itself in all manner of physical symptoms: tense, sore shoulders; headaches; stomach aches; tiredness; and even cramps.

As you exercise you will discover your special needs – perhaps your lower back is sore, or one of your shoulders is particularly tense. The 'breathing space' afforded by exercise may even help you to sort out the problem!

Learning to breathe deeply is an essential part of Medau. This has a calming effect – scientific research has shown that as part of a relaxation programme it can contribute to lowering blood pressure. You will find that as you incorporate the breathing techniques shown in the Art of Energy you will sleep much better at night: compare it with the quality of sleep after a day when you have not exercised.

Because Medau is all-absorbing you will only gradually notice how it applies to everyday life: by learning to manage your body in the most natural and easy way your complex lives will become less stressful.

You do not have to be especially gifted to follow the Art of Energy. You will not be learning something alien, this is the way your body 'wants' to be.

General Benefits to Health

Bodies are built to move – and moving in a way which is correct for the body is best of all. Hinrich Medau was years ahead of his time in monitoring his students' general health. Fitness and health were always considered together and no concessions were ever made to quick fitness goals at the expense of long-term general health.

Today no one would question the benefit of exercise to the body systems. These can be summarized as:

1 Skeleto-muscular System

The skeleton provides the scaffolding for the body. It consists of a framework of bones and cartilages which support the body weight, protect vital organs and provide levers for the muscles to move. Exercise strengthens the bone mass by increasing its density and calcium content; at the same time muscles are toned and strengthened and the joints remain fully mobile.

2 *Cardio-vascular System*

The heart is a muscle which needs to be strengthened through exercise. Raising the heart rate increases the efficiency of the heart muscle, so that with each stroke or contraction there is an increased volume of blood being pushed through the system, making more blood available to the body so as to improve circulation.

Efficient circulation keeps blood vessels elastic and less prone to atheroma (laying down of fat inside vessel walls) which in turn avoids increased blood pressure or more serious heart disease. Good circulation maintains capillaries (the tiniest blood vessels) and can even increase their number; it also maintains the speed and efficiency at which oxygen is taken up by the body. Because blood sustains, feeds and removes toxins from the entire body, the excellent working of the cardio-vascular system is vital.

3 *Nervous System*

The nervous system is extremely complex. There are two main nervous systems: a) the central nervous system which involves the brain and the spinal cord; and b) the peripheral nervous system, a network of nerves which connect the central nervous system with other parts of the body.

Exercise provides both systems with a plentiful supply of blood so that impulses travel to and from the brain into the spinal cord in order to activate muscles and understand sensations.

Command signals from the brain can be sent out by two pathways: the somatic system which triggers contractions under the brain's conscious control, i.e. all the movements you choose to do; and the autonomic system, which triggers reactions and functions of smooth muscles unconsciously, or involuntarily, such as the workings of the heart, lungs and stomach.

Exercise affects the nervous system in other ways too: a strong back will protect the spinal cord by preventing the likelihood of nerve injury. Training in movement increases all brain activity, including the memory, and speeds up responses and reflexes. Finally, it calms and clears the mind.

4 Respiratory System

This is the system which makes oxygen available to the body, involving the lungs, air passages and the diaphragm. The latter is a large band of muscle attached to the ribs: it contracts spontaneously, acting like a pair of bellows which draw air into the lungs. Like all muscles it is made more efficient through exercise, achieving maximum air capacity and thus making more oxygen available to the body. The action of the diaphragm is said to affect the inner organs such as the liver and stomach through the 'breathing wave'. The elasticity of the intercostal muscles, which run between the ribs, also affects the expansion of the lungs.

Oxygen is the vital element to human life which converts food into energy: it is often referred to as the body fuel. It is breathed in, taken into the lungs and transported by single-cell air sacs (alveoli) into the capillaries. At the same time carbon dioxide is passed from the capillaries into the air sacs to be breathed out. The oxygen is then transported through the circulatory system to wherever it is needed.

5 Digestive System

This involves the taking in and absorption of food. After passing through the mouth, mixing with saliva, the food passes down the oesophagus into the stomach, where it is mixed with gastric juices, broken down and partly absorbed. It passes into the small intestine by peristaltic waves where most of the absorption takes place through the intestinal walls. It is absorbed partly into the blood system and partly into the lymphatus (mainly fats). Then the food mass moves into the large intestine where much of its fluid is reabsorbed and the waste is evacuated.

By improving the circulation, exercise aids peristalsis and good digestion and speeds up a sluggish metabolism – the rate at which the food is used by the body. Exercise is also clinically proven to have good effects on eating disorders: whether this is purely psychological, or whether it actually balances trace elements in the blood, thought to affect anorexia and bulimia, is not yet known.

6 Lymphatic System

This consists of a network of vessels or canals like small veins which carry body fluid – seeped from the capillaries – back up through the body to the main large veins. Throughout the lymphatic canals there are small valves which control the flow of the lymph fluid, preventing it from running backwards. The onward passage of the fluid is caused by the external pressure of surrounding muscles. Good muscle tone and regular muscular contraction affect this movement like a pump.

The lymphatic system also contains a series of vitally important glands, or nodes, which manufacture lymphocytes, one of the five forms of white cell which play a critical role in the body's system of defence against disease.

It has been found that the spring or rebound with the moment of weightlessness (see the Development of Medau, page 22) has a strong, stimulating effect on the lymphatic canals. Effective lymphatic drainage prevents a leaden feeling in your legs (pooling), puffy ankles, and helps to prevent cellulite.

7 Health and Vitality

Recent clinical evidence suggests that strong rhythmic movements – done continuously – can relieve pre-menstrual symptoms and painful periods (dysmenorrhoea). This is because continuous exercise is thought to release endorphins, a group of chemicals which scientists believe have pain-relieving properties. Little is known about endorphins but some feel that they have a role in regulating body heat, respiration, eating, learning, sexual behaviour and the control of the heart and blood vessels.

It has been suggested that a combination of oxygen and endorphins produces that feeling of well-being you experience after exercising. Evidently further research on endorphins is needed but the old adage of 'walking away the blues' seems now to have some scientific basis.

Also there is no doubt that complexions are improved with exercise. Sweating expels toxins through the skin so that it is cleansed more thoroughly: keep to a regular exercise regime and you will notice that your complexion becomes clearer, more translucent. The increased blood supply is essential in keeping muscles toned so that the overlying skin is smoother and literally blooms.

8 Medau for Your Back: A Special Mention

Think of the spine, plus the spinal cord which runs through the column of the vertebrae, as something like the spine of a book. It quite literally connects and holds the body together.

All nerve impulses 'fly' up and down the cord to and from the brain. Not only that. *Every* muscle in the body is connected, either directly or indirectly, to the spine. This means that every movement we make refers to the back in some way.

More than 80 per cent of people over the age of thirty suffer from varying degrees of back pain and the problem seems to be getting more widespread. Pain is the body's warning signal that all is not well.

WHY ARE OUR BACKS SO VULNERABLE?

The spine consists of 25 separate cube-like bones called vertebrae. Lighter and smaller at the top and increasing in size in the lower/middle back (lumbar area) these vertebrae stack up in a long curving column like cotton reels on a string, which supports the weight of the entire upper body. This is no mean feat. The body weight is carried down into the five fused vertebrae of the sacrum which makes up part of the pelvis.

Complex sets of ligaments and muscles which attach to the vertebrae allow the spine to bend forwards (forward flexion), backwards (lateral flexion) and rotate (twist).

Seen from the side the spine has natural curves which act as springs, absorbing some of the impact of the body weight on the ground. These curves are named as specific areas of the spine, each with slightly different characteristics and different degrees of mobility. Starting at the top:

1   Seven vertical vertebrae support the head and neck. The top two, the atlas and axis, allow the head to rotate.
2   Twelve thoracic vertebrae form the area of the spine to which the twelve pairs of ribs are attached. They do not move much as they support and

protect the lungs, heart and other vital organs. The spine curves outwards at this point and can become prone to 'hoop' back; this is not surprising considering most people spend much of their time bending forward. There is a constant need to pull up and straighten this part of the back.

3　Five lumbar vertebrae carry the main weight of the body. They are the largest vertebrae and, although placed between the fairly fixed thoracic vertebrae and the solid sacrum, they are very mobile. The large iliopsoas muscles which help to hold the pelvis in place are attached to these vertebrae. There is a lot of strain and tension in this area which is very prone to pain and injury. The lumbar vertebrae are often said to be 'overworked and underpaid'.

4　Five fused vertebrae of the sacrum form part of the pelvis. They disperse the body weight outwards and down into the legs. The coccyx, or vestigial tail, has very little purpose, except for providing an attachment for part of the pelvic floor.

DISCS

Between the vertebrae, keeping them separate, are gelatinous discs or cushions of soft cartilage which are elastic and add mobility to the spine. These discs make up about one-third of the length of the spine and act as shock absorbers between the vertebrae. When you are standing, the discs are compressed; when you lie down and take the pressure off your back they reshape like a sponge resuming its shape after being squeezed. Movement, too, stimulates the discs and keeps them 'plump' and the vertebrae intact.

Discs can, unfortunately, 'slip' all too easily, although this is an inaccurate description: it means they get damaged, or herniate, so that they bulge out and sometimes expose their softer gelatinous centre which can press on nerves and cause muscle spasm. A major cause of back strain, this condition is dangerous and painful. The accident-prone lumbar spine is most vulnerable to disc problems.

SPINAL CORD

Running through and protected by the vertebrae is the spinal cord.

This elongated bundle of nerve tracts is very vulnerable to the vagaries of the vertebrae. Any misalignment of the spine (or disc bulge) can trap or press the nerves, causing intense pain which can be referred to other parts of the body.

With highly complex sets of muscles and ligaments holding erect an essentially unstable column of bones, the whole of the spinal column looks potentially like a disastrous piece of design. In addition to the potential weaknesses, it has been said that standing erect is the back's first and main problem. Humans as a species have grown too tall and too heavy for a spine whose design was originally intended for four-footed movement. We are constantly battling against the pull of gravity while perched on two small feet – dispersing the weight on all fours would probably be safer!

Our backs perform, therefore, a suprising balancing act. But the problem is that bodies are rarely symmetrical. Even slight variations in the length of legs or strength of one side of the body (the favoured right or left) can cause long-term postural injuries and back pain.

Few of us escape falls, injuries and accidents, and these inevitably adversely affect the back. It is a sad fact that not enough people can take the time to recover. We are all guilty of making sudden and unexpected demands on our backs, so always think again before embarking on something entirely new – beware of DIY books which tell you how to erect a garage in an afternoon! Be realistic about your strength: heaving suitcases, shovelling snow, pushing the car, or simply standing too long on high heels, can all affect your back.

STRESS MANAGEMENT

Anxiety and stress are frequently registered in our backs. Clenched teeth and tension in the neck can cause painful spasm. If you have severe or recurring back pain or obvious abnormal curvature of the spine (scoliosis, kyphosis or lordosis) consult your doctor immediately.

The first step to back care is sensible maintenance. Experts can be consulted who will check your environment to see that working surfaces, car seats, wash basins and cupboards are correctly placed for you.

Try to be aware of anything which might be aggravating your back. Are you, for instance, sitting sensibly with your body straight and your feet uncrossed? Do you carry heavy shopping frequently? What is your position when sitting at a desk? An illustration of the importance of these questions is an acquaintance of mine whose neck became locked on one side. Her physiotherapist pointed out that this was exactly the position in which she sat all day with the telephone tucked under her chin.

The Stretch section in the Art of Energy workout is perfect for the back. Start by 'balancing' the head, stretching the neck, flattening the thoracic spine and easing out the lumbar area. Posture checks and the strengthening and mobilizing movements on the floor (when the spine is supported) complete the package.

Medau is especially good for backs because:

1 The strain or effort of movement is dispersed correctly through your whole back. No one part is overstrained. Muscles are worked rhythmically without jarring or jolting the joints. This cuts out wear and tear and achieves great economy of effort.

2 Muscles retain their youthful tone and elasticity so that they fully support your back. The abdominals are strengthened in harmony with your back muscles, creating a strong elastic girdle to support the vulnerable lumbar spine.

3 Your body is always in perfect alignment and never distorted from its natural shape. The long, elastic 'through' body stretches ease out your back muscles, freeing and pulling the vertebrae back into correct alignment.

4 You will achieve a strength and resilience which maximizes your body's natural rebound. By taking the weight upwards, the lightness in the chest relieves the overworked lumbar spine.

5 The many changes of weight, dynamic or effort in the movements ensures that the whole muscle is used to its full potential, not just strengthened in uneven patches.

6 Your body will be long and lithe, not overbulky and heavy, which places the strain of extra weight on the back. Over-

developed muscles, such as the shoulders, can impede the free movements of joints.

7 All the natural movements of the spine are practised slowly and with care. Your back is educated into an unconscious awareness of how to move with strength and safety. This helps to avoid the long-term stresses and daily mishaps which cause so much pain and inconvenience.

Nothing is more ageing and more inhibiting than the proverbial bad back. Much can be done through a little care and correct management.

No one should underestimate the surge of *confidence* which regular exercise brings through better body shape, improved skin condition and the feeling of optimism and well-being. Movement and exercise are crucial to general health, not just as preventative medicine, but as a step towards assuming responsibility and control over your life.

5 *The Way a Class Works*

I have been asked 'What can I expect from a Medau class?' and 'How is Medau different from other exercise movements?' This chapter explains the concept of 'movement technique' which Lala and I apply to all our teaching.

Hinrich Medau saw 'rhythmic movement' as only part of a comprehensive teacher training course replacing the traditional free standing exercises. In Medau's hands it became a brilliant tool to display his work. He found that, over the years, it provided an excellent basic body training which seemed to underpin and support all their other studies in athletics and dance. There were fewer injuries amongst the students, and they coped far better with the work load of the course.

The Medau body is a body which lasts – witness the fact that together with many other Medau teachers I am still trim and teaching full time

after forty years! This is why, with our longer life expectancy and the great variety of roles we are all asked to play in contemporary life, Medau produces the ideal body shape (see page 30).

Medau applied his movement training technique to students who were already unusually fit and heavily programmed into the set forms and rules of PE training. He matched this free movement with a freer, more creative, improvized teaching style. Everything had to be fresh and spontaneous, tailor-made for a particular group at a particular time. This was a totally new approach to teaching, which left a great deal to the inspiration and flair of the individual psyche. Very few rules were laid down and guidelines only were given on class structure.

Slowly over the years a pattern has emerged which, with considerable concessions to changes of pace and style, is still the basis of our improvized teaching today. This pattern has been applied to the video and the book. The Art of Energy routines are but a starting point.

It is a challenge to teach 'intuitively' and this is one reason why I enjoy teaching 'movement'. It is stimulating and rewarding, and a chance, as someone said, 'to teach without brakes'.

One question I'm constantly asked about teaching is, 'But how is it done?' I have based the design of the Art of Energy programme on Medau's basic teaching principles:

1   You need to start with the body – all the movements are based on a sound knowledge of physiology and anatomy plus a practical grasp of how the body actually works (there is more about this on page 34).

2   You need to have someone really good to guide you. Follow Lala carefully. You need to get the 'look' or correct body image firmly in your mind to use it as a blueprint for your own movement. If you are watching the video, make sure you follow Lala's rhythm, and if you are

working from the book be sure to follow a rhythm of your own. In class an uneven rhythm always comes over like someone singing off key in a choir.

3   Posture is important. The movement should 'flow through your body'. Ease out stiff joints and try to feel motivated and confident.

4   Rhythm is the great motivator and driving force, and the subtle use of changes of pace and emphasis are vital ways of altering and improving your movement. Pacing yourself correctly is an acquired skill. You need to be very intuitive and respond to your own special needs.

5   Medau classes are structured around what we call movement 'themes'. These might be rhythmics, travelling technique (walking, running, skipping, etc) posture, body alignment, balance (see fitness factors, page 29). In addition to these, the Art of Energy incorporates fitness themes such as swing, spring, balance, care of the back.

6   I always say to people, 'start where you are'. Everyone can move in some way, so begin

where you can manage happily, and never impose a form on your body which feels alien or uncomfortable. Wait for the movement to develop. In one sense, I think that Medau is a matter of setting up situations where the body finds its own best way.

7   When teaching a class we make as few verbal corrections as possible. Movement should be allowed to develop naturally through using other 'corrective' movements. Words are a different idiom and may provoke a false response, e.g. 'Bend your knees a little more' can become an exaggerated self-conscious jerk.

8   The music you use should never be for background, but it should make a vital contribution. As we have seen, rhythm is the driving force behind good movement, supporting and altering it with subtle changes of shape and emphasis. Medau teachers originally accompanied their students on the piano and other percussive instruments. Today the clever use of taped music grows out of this interesting approach.

9   Swinging is very important in Medau for it illustrates clearly the analysis of movement (see page 23). Swinging uses all the large muscle groups in harmony and allows complete coordination, pushing the movement through the pelvis and thrusting the body towards and away from gravity. It provides the strongest way in which the body can function; it is truly the basis of all working movements and will help improve everything from swinging a tennis raquet to throwing a javelin.

10 Great importance is given to springing or rebounding, another basic theme much practised by the early Medau teachers which has the same movement analysis as swinging. Rebounding is the body's natural shock absorber (see page 81). Be sure that in walking, running, skipping and springing every movement has this resilient, springy quality.

11 Don't force your breathing. It needs to be synchronized and in complete harmony with the movement – the ultimate in total coordination.

12 In addition to the fitness factors

(see page 29), 'movement factors' have to be considered when structuring a class. These are:

i Use of space:
Spatial awareness is very important. In thinking about movement, feel that you can use the space freely. Don't remain rooted to the spot. Think of the space around and above you and feel confident about using the whole space.

ii Changes of movement 'dynamic':
Variety and change are the essence of Medau. Vary the rhythm and pace to make your workout stimulating and interesting and try out combinations of fast, slow, heavy and light movements. It adds excitement and variety and will use all parts of the muscle, not just the same 'patches'.

iii Correct body alignment:
Try to keep your movement 'pure'. Medau very much disliked what he called 'affectation' or posing in movement, which he felt disturbed the rhythm and flow of energy. I remember that he used to call loudly to the class 'I want no Baroque twirls, please.'

Purity of line, perfect balance and keeping the body correctly aligned are very important. The ancient Chinese 'meridians' or energy lines form the basis of our breathing and stretching exercises (see page 62). Practise them, as a source of energy to relate the body both to itself and to space.

13 Coordination is important. Try to discover what you feel about movement. I'm always struck with the way some people take to Medau with such astonishing ease. It is as though they have never lost their early natural movement patterns. Others seem to struggle either through having been already programmed into more rigid movement disciplines or, more frequently, because 'letting go' is alien to their basic natures. The release or 'free float' of natural movement can seem baffling to some. They conceive movement as 'conscious' action, whereas the centre of deep rhythmical coordination is completely unconscious and requires no thought.

There have been many magical moments when I have

watched the transition made from conscious to unconscious control. It is like the breaking of an iron barrier: the body rhythm is 'unblocked' and the release and pleasure of natural movement are experienced for the first time.

14 Individualism – movement should be a form of self-expression. Hinrich Medau said 'Only you can get it right.' Nothing is ever imposed from the outside: individual body shape, character, circumstance and taste are totally valid in considering that movement is an 'expression of the self'. Medau produces no clones, but 'whole people' with the confidence and self-respect to be themselves.

15 Every time you practise Medau you should treat it as a unique occasion with a real inner life of its own. You will find that your body feels different on every occasion, even when the workout remains the same. Enjoy and respond to your intuitive body sense. Getting it right for yourself can be an extravagant pleasure. Medau Magic in full force.

Between us, Lala and I teach a tremendous range of classes, applying Medau techniques in many ways and spheres: to toddlers and 'minders'; the under 5s; fitness classes; movement technique classes; one-to-one private teaching; to groups of all ages and in circumstances as varied as Holloway Prison, a drug rehabilitation centre and trendy dance studios.

Teaching a theatre group in New York we worked on movement dynamics, without music, and greatly improved the scope and range of the actors' actions.

Our courses run internationally, covering a wide range of topics including movement technique, rhythmics, fitness, dance motif, choreography, pedagogics and special needs such as children, the elderly and the handicapped. Everything we do is rooted in Medau's original concept of teaching to achieve 'dynamic whole body movement'.

I sometimes use hand apparatus in class. There was and is a very particular way of using hand apparatus (props) in Medau. It should never be used for juggling tricks or simply to decorate the movement, but can be used to intensify the 'through body swing'.

I have to say that in classes which are an hour's fitness package in a dance studio, it is neither safe nor helpful to use props. There is neither time nor space, but the creative use of props is enormously helpful in teaching children and other groups with special needs.

Medau has stood the test of time. It works, and will continue to fill people's lives with light and pleasure.

The Art of Energy

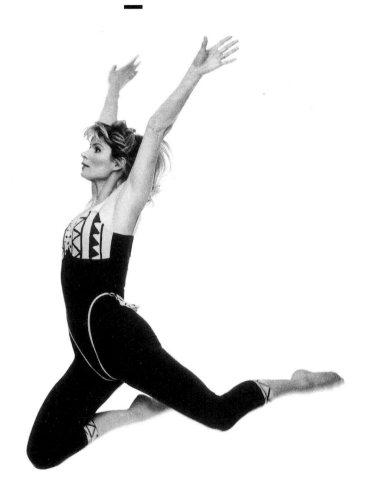

6 *Using the Art of Energy*

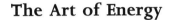

The Art of Energy

This is not a crash course in fitness, but an on-going benefit which will help you to get the best out of yourself. Medau and good movement are sustaining and you will find not only that you will want to return to the Art of Energy again and again but also that you will gradually find yourself applying the principles of good movement to all your activities.

When I was a child my piano teacher would say, 'Only practice makes perfect. If you are not improving you are slipping backwards.' Not so with Medau. Once you have learned the right way to move, the body seems to take over, and daily movements become part of the continuing fitness programme.

Life today has become complex and women, especially, have many roles to play. Each of us needs a strong, reliable, working body, a calm clear mind and endless vitality. Try the Art of Energy now: the perfect programme for the woman of the 90s.

How to Use the Programme

To get the most from this programme, you need to adopt a flexible approach and make it work for you. Remember that fitness is relative to your lifestyle: you should have some clear idea of what you want to be fit for, and what you want the programme to achieve for you.

You can do the four sections – Stamina, Strength, Suppleness and Stretch – in different combinations, depending on how much time you have, and on how you feel. But first, if you have any doubts about your general health and fitness, or if you think you might be overweight or have not exercised for many years, consult your doctor before embarking on the programme.

Here are some suggested variations:

1 The full one-hour programme three times a week, with free days in between. For example, Monday, Wednesday and Saturday. (This is best enjoyed by using the Art of Energy video.)

2 Any combination of two sections such as Strength with Stamina or Strength with Suppleness. Aim to do this five times a week, with an occasional free day in between. For example, Monday, Tuesday, Thursday and all four sections on the Saturday.

3 One section every day – but do not do the same one each time.

4 For a more gradual approach, you could start by trying one section two to three times a week for two weeks, adding an extra section within three weeks. Remember to slow down if you feel it is too much at first, but do not be lazy – it is always easier to decide not to take action! Slowly build the sections up until you have found a level that suits you. You may devise a system which is somewhere between all three of the above.

Do not cheat by doing only your favourite section. The programme is devised as an inter-related package, and the best results require each part to be done equally.

You will need to start with your own, or the set five-minute Warm Up section every time you begin so that muscles and tendons are not pulled. A warm shower, however, will do before Section Four, Suppleness.

More is not necessarily better. The Programme must fit in with and support your lifestyle – it should not become an additional chore. Making time is often the most difficult thing to do at the beginning, but even if you are the busiest person in the world there will always be time for this programme – after all, each section is under 15 minutes in length.

Do not be discouraged if you miss a day – be relaxed and, if you can, make up the time: there is no point in getting despondent if sometimes your plans go awry. If you get bored with the idea of exercising at the same time each day then vary the times of day. The beauty of the Art of Energy is that it is adaptable and flexible, to mirror you and your life.

Choose the sections that best suit your next activity. Do not do Stamina when you want to settle down to sleep or look pale and romantic. It would be better to choose Suppleness on its own. On the other hand, Suppleness alone is not the right preparation for a squash match, where you need Strength and Stamina.

Find the time of day when your energy level is good – not, for example, after a large dinner. Some people find the best time of day to exercise is just after they wake up in the morning: a workout makes them feel more alert, bright and toned before beginning their day. It might seem hard, dragging yourself out of the warm bed – but the benefits are untold.

An excellent time for exercising is early evening when you feel exhausted after a hard day and want to do nothing but flop in front of the television: a strong, warming and invigorating workout can be the very best way to brighten you up for the rest of the evening – the difference can be dramatic – and it will help you sleep better too.

Early evenings are not always good for young mothers: choose a time when your baby is sleeping, perhaps early afternoon, when you are certain you will not be disturbed by other children or partners.

Another tip: resting with your feet up for ten minutes before you begin can help you get your breath.

Starting Points

Here are a few points to bear in mind before starting the programme.

1 Wear something comfortable and stretchy, but not dreary. Feel good about your appearance even if there is no one to see you. Get yourself organized and prepared to begin. (I always start by washing my feet!)

2 Do not force yourself at any time. It spoils the movement and you will probably focus on the wrong muscles. Each movement is carefully designed so that by the end of the session you will have worked all the muscles in your body. Allow your body to find its own way, experiment to begin with and do your own version – perhaps just feet at first, for example, when a movement sequence seems complicated – until you are skilled and strong enough for the real thing.

3 Recognise that performance varies with mood and circumstance. As living beings humans must not lose their intuitive understanding of what is best for them at any given moment. Aim, however, for some level of consistency. One day of hectic enthusiasm followed by three in the doldrums is less effective than four days of more moderate and consistent effort.

4 Think of your body as a whole and aim to move in one piece. You should move without jolting and jerking, with an equal tension through the body, rather like a piece of stretched elastic. You need to balance out the strong, heavy lower body with the lightness of your chest and arms.

The movement must flow through the pelvis, tapping into the energy centre of the body. I think of this as 'Earth energy', as the centre of gravity and also as the body's engine. The chest is light and full of air: I see this as 'Space energy' which carries us upwards away from the earth and into contact with the rest of life. It helps to understand, too, that all movement combines these two: the strong impulse (Earth energy), flowing into the easy 'free float' (Space energy) which prepares for the next strong movement impulse.

Try to think of and feel the movement as growing naturally from deep inside the body – rather like breathing. This is what is called 'organic' movement and gives a sensation of great ease; one movement passes to the next in perfect coordination. It is the reason for the unparalleled safety record of Medau – you simply cannot hurt yourself if you are moving in a way which is right for your body.

5 Unless you are told specifically to breathe out strongly, for instance, when doing abdominal exercises, do not force the breathing patterns or hold your breath. The inner breathing movement will become synchronized and in perfect harmony, leaving mind and body refreshed and unstressed.

6 Do not waft or flop about when exercising. Always keep your body in readiness for the next movement. This is called maintaining minimal muscle tone and supports the skeleton, keeping the body poised for action. You need to be like a cat that can jump with dazzling ease out of deep sleep, to be ready for life's emergencies.

7 Keep well within your limits at the beginning so that you have something to spare. A simple rule is to ensure that you can manage to return to your starting position with relative ease. Try to balance out movements by stretching out then contracting inwards, or by pushing then pulling. Never make a frantic or over-ambitious movement which pushes you to the point of no return and forces you to flop instead of recover. This can be dangerous and damaging to the body. The safest movement is strong, harmonious and totally in control.

Now have fun and love every minute of it.

7 Warm Up

TIME: 5 MINUTES
MUSIC: MEDIUM PACED DISCO WITH A STRONG RHYTHMICAL BEAT

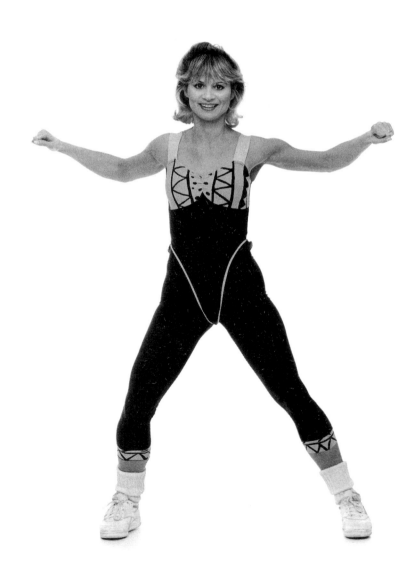

Reasons to Warm Up

The body functions best when it is warm. Muscles become more pliable and less prone to injury and joints are more mobile. The lungs expand more easily, increased oxygen is made available, circulation improves, toxins and waste products are dispersed more efficiently. Warmth is the body's signal to go. Think of a hibernating bear waiting to stir in the spring sunshine.

Shoes are optional if you have a good springy surface, but it is essential to keep feet and ankles warm. Use the floor as a spring board, moving out of the floor, not into it. Disperse the impact through the body, using and not impairing the body's natural spring.

Put on the music and feel the beat, or sing and hum in marching time. Think of the rhythm as a strong driving force and allow it to push you along. Feel the earth rhythm under your feet strengthening and motivating you.

The Movements

1 Begin with heel presses and arm swings. Standing well balanced with feet hip width apart, keeping your toes down, alternately press and lift heels, remaining on the spot. Make sure you step with equal weight on each foot, and that there is no favoured leg. This warms the feet and lower legs, especially the Achilles tendon. Swing your arms in time with the music, moving the opposite arm and leg forwards and backwards in time with your steps.

2 Get the breathing going and lift your elbows slightly as you swing. Now lift your feet so that you are actually marching, making sure you are using the upper leg muscles. Stretch out both arms and slowly raise them to your sides and up above your head. This eases the body upwards against gravity and stimulates the diaphragm. Feel free to open your mouth and yawn, which will release any tension in your neck. Slowly lower your arms. Repeat at least four times.

3   Move into side steps. Step to one side and bring the other foot across to meet it. Step, together, left and right, bringing the body weight across. Think of the movement as 'step and together, step and together'. Bend your knees slightly as your foot moves sideways. This warms up the inner and outer leg muscles. You should aim to repeat this eight times, then another eight times.

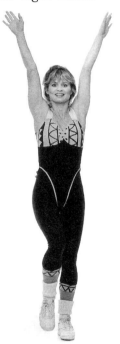

4   Now go back to marching on the spot with increased effort. It's all to do with warming the legs and body.

5   Repeat arm stretches slowly and strongly. Move your arms as if they are wings that grow out of the torso (upper body), rather than just attachments from the shoulder. Feel the movement warming and activating your chest and back muscles. Deepen your breathing.

6   Repeat the side steps (16 times), then go into double side steps. Step left-together, left-together and back again, then step right-together, right-together. Lift your knees slightly and swing your arms vigorously out and in, keeping your elbows bent. Try clapping your hands together on the second step, warming your hands as you enjoy the rhythm.

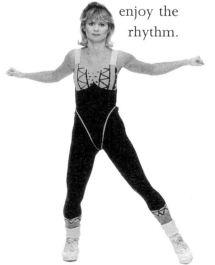

7 Scoots and tugs are strong, short pulls and punches with your arms to the left and right. They should be fun and make you feel considerably warmer.

TUGS

Tug fists vigorously towards hips with your weight on the opposite leg (two on each side for 16 counts). Find and use the energy around the pelvic area. Do not wiggle – these pelvic movements should be small and strong, keeping the body held strongly in correct tension.

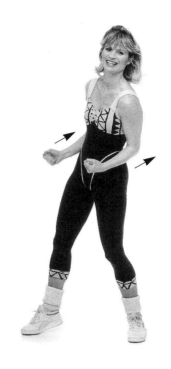

SCOOTS

Make small punches away from your body at shoulder level (two on each side for 16 counts). Keep neck and upper back in strong and correct tension. Be careful not to whip your neck backwards and forwards.

   Repeat the tugs and scoots alternately.

8 Take the stepping into jogging forwards and backwards or move around the room to relieve the pressure on your feet (32 times).

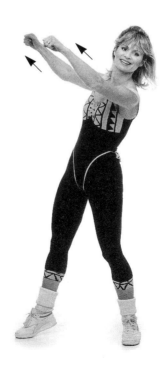

9 Jog on the spot and repeat the slow arm lifts. Carry the body weight high and remember the body's natural spring.

10 Repeat side steps and double side steps, then go back to jogging.

11 Release the feet in small alternate forward kicks. Enjoy feeling light and springy and avoid the feeling of leaden feet.

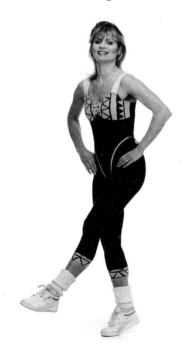

12 Stand with your feet apart and swing your hips from side to side in time to the music. This is very rhythmical. It is called zagging, and relieves the lower

back. Do not flop, or lock the knees, but feel strong and elastic.

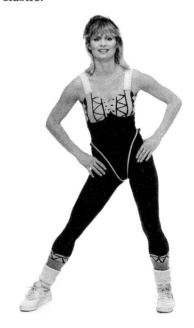

13 Return to jogging, moving about freely and changing direction if you wish, or run forwards and backwards if there is enough space. Improvize your own steps if you wish. Be as exotic or as everyday as you wish. Your energy levels should be high.

You should now feel warmed and thoroughly motivated to carry on. Don't be tempted to pause or sit down at this point. Keep moving, however gently, before going on to the next section.

8 *Stretch: the Energy of Water*

TIME: 12 MINUTES
MUSIC: SLOW

Why We Need to Stretch

Stretching is one of the most natural and necessary of human movements. Lala's programme will show you how to develop good posture and avoid back problems. (See also Medau for backs page 38.) Stretching will help:

1 To restore the length of the muscles which shorten during rest. That's why we like to stretch in bed in the morning, easing out the tug of shortened muscles and tendons.

2 To counter the force of gravity which implodes our bodies, setting up pressures on joints and internal organs.

3 To correct and compensate for occupational hazards.

We spend so much time slumped over one task or another and too much time sitting on chairs.

4 To deepen our breathing by stimulating the diaphragm – the large domed muscle attached to our ribs that contracts downwards, pulling air into our lungs. This is why stretching and

yawning go together. Breathe freely, but breathe out as you extend, to lengthen the stretch.

How to Stretch

The body, by its natural structure, has invisible lines through which it stretches with greatest effect and and complete safety. We call these correctly aligned stretches, and interestingly they follow the ancient Chinese 'energy lines'. All strong stretches must follow these lines, passing through the body from one point of extremity to the other in a long, smooth stretch without any break in the middle. There should be no points of weakness or collapse, regardless of whether the lines are cross stretches involving twisting, or are pulling out or outward stretches. Stretches should be correctly supported so that you never get to the point of no return. Always retain the feeling of inner support or centring which can pull the body back to the starting pos-ition, often the upright position, or into the equal and opposite stretch passing through the starting position.

Never jab at a stretch, as it will feel like an emergency to the muscle. The stretch reflex, which I call the anti-stretch reflex, will clamp the muscle to prevent a poss-ible injury. This is why bouncing in a stretch is bad, and can be compared to driving a car while applying and releasing the brakes.

There should be no strain, but a feeling of blissful release. Coax and persuade the muscles to stretch. Feel confident and think up, out or across. We say, put your thoughts into the stretch and 'go with it'.

As a movement, stretching has been minutely observed and analyzed and various types of stretch have been postulated. In Medau we tend to think in terms of changing the pace and weight of the stretch. Some are more sustained and are held in extension for longer than others to allow for increased stretching. We keep the feeling of a living, dynamic two-way movement full of elasticity and strength, refreshing and renewing itself.

The Movements

Preparing the back
It is vital to take care of the back, since all major muscle groups attach

to it in some way. The back muscles should hang downwards from the shoulders, like a coat on a hanger. The back is divided into three sections: upper, middle and lower. The upper/middle back is particularly difficult to exercise because it is fairly rigid. It is known as the wasteland of the upper back. The lower back is the hollow of the back. It takes much of the weight of the body. Although it is a natural and necessary curve, it can become exaggerated and strained.

1   Stand with feet hip width apart. Feel long and extended through your back and neck. This is your posture line. Start from the top and focus on each area of the spine so that you work down through the whole of your back. To help you achieve this, imagine a line going up the spine and through the crown of your head.

2   Gently turn your head from side to side, freeing the neck. When it is correctly balanced your head should feel very light.

3   Tilt your head forwards and press gently, stretching the back of the neck while rounding the whole back, then return to the vertical.

4   Check your posture by lightly placing your hands on the top of your head (a), then on your shoulders (b), checking that they are not hunched, and then

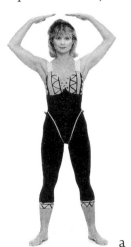
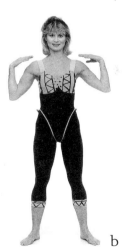
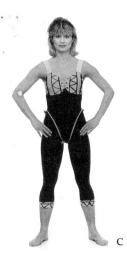

a   b   c on your hips (c), checking that they are level. In this position you are correctly aligned, and are balanced in 'vertical' extension. The least amount of energy is required to remain upright.

5 Repeat the movement outlined in (3), with a deeper bend, slowly breathing out to empty your lungs, then breathing in strongly through your nose. Wait for the 'turning point', when inhale becomes exhale, and try to feel the deep breath inside your body. This will increase the amount of oxygen in the body and will help you to find extra energy to support and sustain the movements.

6 Circle your arms lightly around your head, lifting the weight upwards from the chest which is the body's 'centre of lightness'. If you think upwards, the movement will feel easy – we say, 'make a balloon and let it rise'. This counters the compressing effect of gravity and helps to realign the spine. It also conserves energy by using the body's natural lightness to take the weight of the upper body well out of the hips.

Take your arms up, keeping the feeling of lightness in your chest.

7 Bend your elbows and flatten the upper back between the shoulder blades. Press the shoulder blades together and then release them, working the wasteland of the upper back. Increase the pressure by dropping your hands behind you and pressing them together. Release and squeeze again.

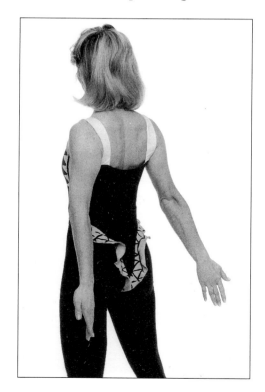

8 Press your hands on your knees, rounding the middle back and tightening the abdominals into the back. Hold the position and strengthen it. Feel firm and strong. Lift the upper body out of the hips, relieving pressure in the lower back.

This combines strengthening the muscles with increasing the suppleness of the spine.

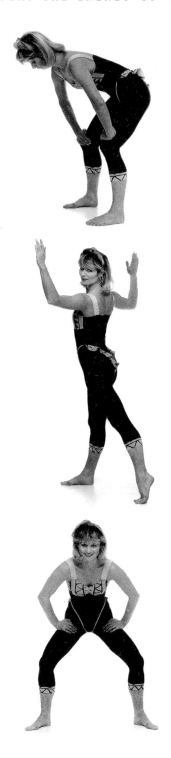

9 Bend your knees, lift your body and press into a side twist. Allow the leg to follow the movement round, so that the body remains aligned. Pull upwards 'out' of the hips, positioning the arms as in the photograph, and repeat left and right.

10 Stand with your feet apart, taking the focus into the base of your spine. Press down into a half squat, dropping the pelvis. Feel as though you are about to sit down. Then pull up strongly through the whole back, tightening the pelvic floor. This is the 'centre of strength' of the body, the centre of gravity where we find the strongest muscles and the highest internal

pressure. Pull the strength and energy up from the ground, feeling the natural strength of the whole body and allowing it to flow upwards. We are creatures of earth and air, rooted to the ground but suspended in space.

11 This is the St Andrew's Cross (right). Pull outwards with your arms wide, stretching the sides. With your arms and legs in a star shape, feel the stretch crossing through the body. Try to 'go with it' rather than 'for it'.

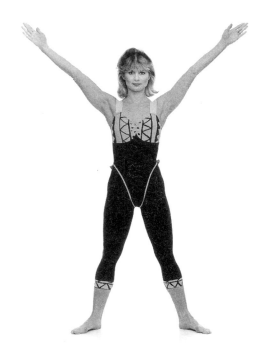

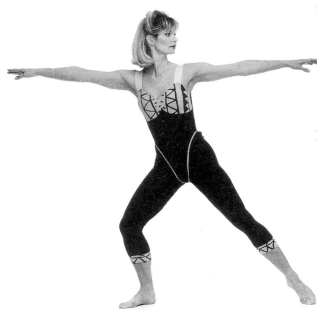

12 Drop your arms to the horizontal. Rock from right to left, reaching out strongly with your hands and arms, feeling the involvement of the back.

13 Raise your arms, pull them down strongly to your sides with fists clenched and feel the spine growing upwards 'through' the arms. There is a tendency to tip the pelvis forwards. A hollow back made worse by wearing high heels does not help. Remind yourself to tuck your bottom under, tilting the pubic bone upwards.

14 Stand with your knees slightly bent and feet hip width apart, with your hands on your hip joints. Now push your hips forwards and release backwards while pulling up from underneath, tightening the muscles of the pelvic floor. Use the energy from this most powerful part of the body. It should be a strong elastic column with abdominals, lower back and gluteus (buttock) muscles working together.

Side stretches

Once the back and abdominals are strong, we can safely move into side stretches. Feel the body opening out and stretching from fingers to feet along safe body lines. All of these stretches pass through and come back to the vertical posture line. They are strong, rhythmical and symmetrical, involving the whole body in a stretch of equal tension, like a piece of elastic. Each outward thrust is compensated for by an equal and opposite stretch. This gives a push and pull effect, swinging from one direction to another with a strong movement through the pelvis.

There should be no jerking or jolting, but strong, smooth, dynamic movement which will gradually increase in strength and extent as the body grows more used to stretching.

15 Stand with your feet apart and, resting your left hand on your knee, lift up your right arm and lean across to the left into a side stretch, making a line from fingertip to toe. Do not push too far, and be certain to feel strong around the abdominals and middle back. Pull the arm back leaning to the left to refresh the stretch. Repeat the stretch four times on the right and then on the left.

16 Now add a twist: push your left arm out across the body level with your shoulder in a twisting motion, relaxing the other arm. Repeat on the other side.

17 Using the first side stretch, lean out further, supporting the body with your left hand on your knee. You should be making a diagonal line from hand to foot. Repeat. Stretch across very strongly then pull the body upwards to the vertical with your right hand. Then repeat the same stretch to the right. Do not exaggerate the stretch, or tilt forwards or backwards, but try to work with one strong, clean pull. Hold for a slow count of eight, then upwards for eight, then across to the other side for eight.

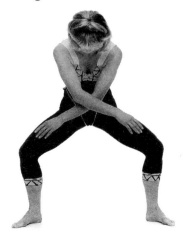

18 Stand upright with your feet apart, distributing the weight evenly and pressing your heels down. Bend your knees and scoop up energy in a strong upward thrust from the feet.

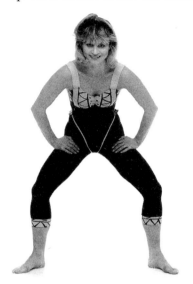

19 Now focus the stretch on the groin and legs. As for exercise 9, stand with your feet apart and press the knees outwards in line with the toes, tilting forwards as you do this. This is a plié. Strengthen your legs by pulling up through the groin and move slowly back to the vertical.

20 Repeat the same knee bends, or pliés, then twist the upper body, taking the leg round (see

exercise 9). This is an easy body twist which it is necessary to follow through. Pull up strongly from the hips and twist the upper body, making sure the leg follows through. The body can move with enormous strength on a natural spiral which takes the strain. This is the basic movement for all ball games and throwing sports.

21 From the vertical, lean the right arm across to the left, supporting the body with your left hand on your knee. Stretch across the bending knee and back to an upright position. Begin by stretching to knee level and gradually pushing down to the floor.

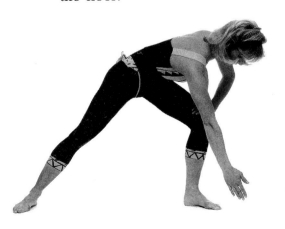

22 Start with your feet slightly apart, with your arms up and outstretched, pulling out from the hips and pressing the heels into the floor. Lean slightly forwards and hold. This is a very strong stretch.

23 Push forwards and down into strong swings, bending your knees and swinging under and up at the back (rebound). Think of reaching up and over as you swing forward. This uses all the muscles, with the whole body in total harmony. Continue with the vertical stretches as a preparation for each swing. Keep your abdominals firm and feel great strength in the back and pelvis.

24 Stretch sideways to flatten and open the back, as in (12). This is a strong movement through the pelvis.

25 Finally, take time to stand and check your posture, and rest and balance in the vertical.

9 *Strength: the Energy of Earth*

TIME: 12–15 MINUTES
MUSIC: STRONG, CLASSICAL

Why We Need to Build Strength

Medau is about building a stronger body. The exercises have been devised to help achieve a lithe shape without developing bulky muscles. The muscles have several important functions. They hold the skeleton in place, take the pressure off the joints and enable the body to cope with life's tasks.

Each strong muscle contraction should be followed by an equally strong stretch, or contra-movement, so that the muscles remain long and elastic rather than becoming chunky. Tightening the muscles strengthens, tones and shapes them. These movements should be done 'in weight', using small but very strong, slow muscular contractions, with variations of effort or pressure. Move slowly, as if working against water, and do not flop or let go of the tension.

Try not to develop patches of strong muscles in the so-called problem areas of abdominals, buttocks and thighs, but involve the whole body, especially the back, distributing the strength evenly throughout.

Bulky muscles can constrain the joints, and too many repetitions of the same movement can actually damage them and lead to long-term injury. They can also impede movement. Overdeveloped muscles such as large thighs or bunched shoulders can become very heavy and inelastic. As you get older these will have a tendency to sag. Medau movement is designed to keep the muscles long and elastic, to avoid stress on the joints and to maintain the body's youthful resilience.

The Movements

1   Make a fist and squeeze it. Feel the muscles harden in your hand and lower arm.

2   Stand with your feet apart and your arms by your sides, palms facing forwards. Bend your arms up in front of you and pull your elbows in towards your body, bending your knees and contracting the abdomen strongly at the same time.

3   Gradually straighten your arms and legs, keeping up the pressure by tightening the buttocks as you pull your body upwards.

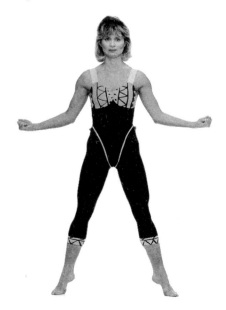

4 Stand in the same position with your arms crossed in front of you. This is known as the 'sumo wrestler'! Then squeeze your elbows together behind you, tightening the upper back, at the same time, straightening the legs.

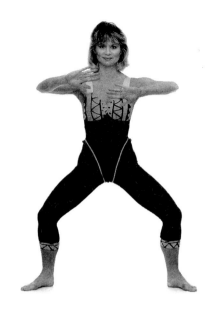

5 Keep your feet apart and push your arms down to the floor with your knees bent, like a weight lifter. Now imagine you are picking up a bar. Heave it up to shoulder level, turn your hands back and thrust it upwards. Use your whole back, tightening the buttocks. Feel the strength and energy in the strongest muscles of the body pushing upwards against gravity.

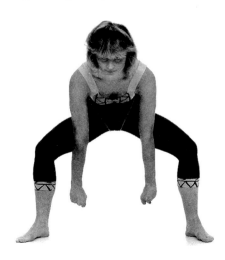

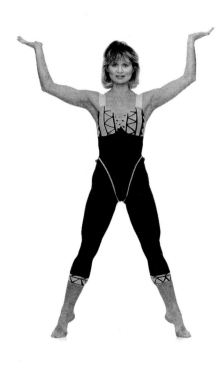

6 Push one arm sideways and
   downwards across the body in a
   strong twist. Pull your shoulders
   up and move both arms behind
   and back, tightening the upper
   back. Repeat with the other side.

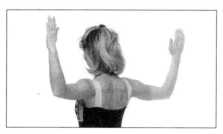

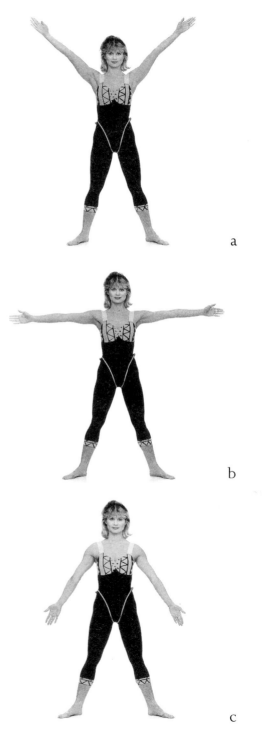

a

7 Adopt the position in exercise 2.
   Contract inwards, then make a
   sharp strong movement outwards using your arms, repeating
   four times. As you pull outwards,
   hold to a count of four, holding
   a strong stretch in each of the
   following breathing positions
   (photographs a, b and c show
   some of the basic lines along
   which the body stretches).

b

8 This movement occurs in the
   stretch section (page 69) to
   mobilize the lower back. Perform
   it now in tension, with a very
   strong forward swing, tightening
   the buttocks and pushing up the
   pelvic floor, then press back.
   The swing goes under, then up,
   then under, then back.

c

9 Reach forward with your arms
and lift them up, then pull out
from your body, as if leaning
forward over a barrel, with your
knees bent. Reach to the floor,
or to knee level

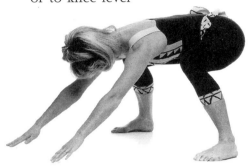

if that is easier for you, and pull
up your whole body, feeling
your whole body weight and
strengthening your legs and
back. Be sure to contract the
abdomen strongly as you do
this, to protect the back. Move
slowly and enjoy the powerful
control of your body weight.

10 Move downwards, controlling
your weight on one knee,
tucking that leg underneath you.
Gently lower your buttocks onto
the floor and bring your knees
up in front of you. Squeeze your
knees up to your chest, pushing
the lower abdomen against the
spine. Keep the pressure up for
at least a count of eight.

11 Place one hand under one knee
and the other hand over it and
hold on. Lean back slowly with
the abdominals held in tightly,
back flattened and buttocks
tight. Change legs and pull up
more strongly with the other
leg. Cross your feet and squeeze
the thighs and pelvic floor,
pushing both heels down. Place
a cushion behind your
back for
more ease.

12 There are specific abdominal
movements involving particular
muscles. As a general rule, blow
out strongly on the muscle
contraction, pulling the
abdominals inwards towards the
spine. Do not pouch the
abdominal muscles as this will
thicken, not flatten the
abdomen.

13 Roll back onto the floor. A
cushion under the lower back
will help beginners. Start with
your knees bent and flatten your
back. Draw your knees up,
contracting the lower
abdominals strongly as you do

this. The lower abdominals are situated just above the pubic bone. Pull up the pelvic floor with strong, slow pulls. Slide your feet along the floor, to give the abdominals a long, strong stretch.

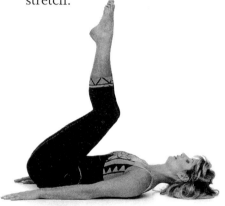

14 Now place a cushion under your head. Bend your knees and raise your upper body, pulling up just enough for your fingers to touch your knees. Support your head with one arm if you need to. These are inward contractions below the ribcage. Stretch out as above when necessary.

15 Combine the movements for the upper and lower abdominals. Raise your knees and squeeze the lower abdominals, then put your feet down and lift the upper body, pulling inwards. Stretch out.

16 From a prone position, pull up, twisting your body to the left, with your knees bent. Flatten your back onto the floor between each lift. Repeat four times to the left and four times to the right.

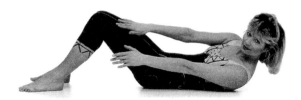

Repeat these lifts to each side of your knees and 'pulse' the movement, or stretch forward. Stretch out.

17 Lie back flat on the floor, then pull up strongly, using your arms and legs, and hold the position for at least a count of eight. Remember to pull the abdominals inwards.

(See facing page)

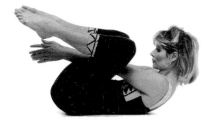

18 Pull up, raising the upper body, then lie back smoothly. Push the pelvis upwards, tighten the thighs and bottom. This lengthens and stretches the rectus abdominus.

19 Sit with your legs in front of you, with one leg stretched out and one bent. Take your weight on both hands and, pressing your heels into the ground, bounce your bottom with very small contractions, raising and lifting off the floor. As an alternative exercise, lean back on your elbows, place a cushion under your middle back and press the weight of your body onto your heels. Contract and release the buttock muscles strongly.

20 Straighten your legs and pull up your legs and your upper body strongly, grasping your right leg with both hands. Feel the tension all the way through your back, abdominals and thighs. Cross your legs and squeeze your thighs as you come up.

For a less strenuous version, place a cushion under your lower back before carrying out the exercise.

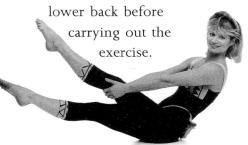

21 Stretch out and roll over onto your front, easing out your neck and shoulders. Keeping your legs long, lift your feet two inches off the floor and 'air walk' slowly in small steps. Bend your knees and squeeze your feet into your bottom. Walk again.

This is extremely strenuous and can be done keeping one leg on the floor and bending the knees alternately. As you get

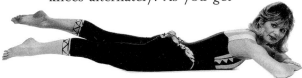

stronger, try lifting your feet with your knees apart. Do not lift your legs too high as you will strain your back.

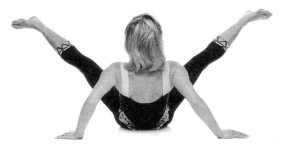

Roll over and push yourself up into the sitting position.

22 Roll back and with your hands supporting your body, swing up into a strong position with your legs extended. This is called a 'half-basket'.

23 Be aware of the weight of your body, roll sideways on to your hands and knees. Bring the right foot forward, then the left, moving into a straight-backed squat. Feel like a weight lifter, and move into a standing position, thrusting your weight upwards, and pulling your arms down.

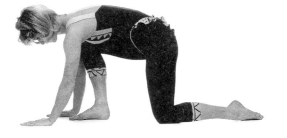

24 Free the neck by gently turning the head from side to side, with the mouth open. Wriggle your shoulders to release the tension.

You have now worked all the main muscle groups, and should feel strong and toned and in touch with your body's muscular energy. Gradually build up the length of time you hold the positions and the number of repetitions. You should feel full of warmth and vitality, strength and confidence. Your body will become more reliable as you develop your strength and endurance.

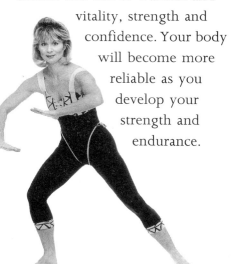

10 *Stamina: the Energy of Fire*

TIME: 15–20 MINUTES
MUSIC: FAST, STRONG BEAT

Why We Need Stamina

Raising the heartbeat, puffing and sweating have become the 'done thing'. Some useful research has been done into the effects of this on the body, and we now know that raising the heart rate within specific limits for at least twenty minutes strengthens the heart muscle, enabling it to operate more efficiently and improve circulation.

This, combined with our knowledge of correct movement, has become the basis of Medau stamina work. It can, therefore, be enjoyable and beneficial for everyone.

Long before the craze for working out to loud music which arrived in the 1970s, we were running, skipping and springing as part of movement classes, and Medau's students were famous for their agility. This was called 'travelling technique' and included many stepping patterns and dances. These could be choreographed into step dance and rhythmic patterns making groupwork more fun by using the space more imaginatively.

The style was strong, springy and

elastic, carrying the body weight easily, and these techniques were used as the starting point for athletics, gymnastics and folk dance. Strength, endurance, agility, coordination and spring were the main aims. With the increased interest in stamina in the 1980s, these techniques have assumed new importance.

How to Move Correctly

Stamina work can become an uncomfortable chore if performed repetitively. It should always be fun, so that you are able to motivate yourself without becoming bored. Medau uses rhythm and music in an interesting and varied way, which helps to make stamina work seem easy.

Be sure that you work at your own pace, so that you feel comfortable the whole time. Ease yourself into it, then increase the pace when you feel ready. Use a variety of steps and vary the impact of the steps you use, so that the weight comes down on a different part of the foot each time. This disperses the weight and helps prevent injury.

As your coordination improves you will be able to try ever more complicated steps. Try to become aware of the space around you, and use it by moving in different directions forwards and backwards, sideways and turning and by making different body shapes.

The Movements

The following points are guidelines for safe stamina work. You will find suggested exercises at the end of this chapter.

Shoes must be worn for the stamina section. You may notice that Lala is not wearing shoes for some of the jumps. This is for demonstration only, and is not advisable unless you are extremely agile and/or well trained.

1 Start by thinking about your posture. Remind yourself of how to do this by looking back to page 63. Ease out the neck and shoulders. Balance your body evenly between your feet, carrying the weight upwards and remembering the centre of lightness in the chest. Keep the body held firmly, paying special attention to holding your spine correctly.

2 Use your body's natural spring and your feet like shock absorbers so that you are rebounding rather than hitting the floor like a hammer. This rebounding stimulates lymphatic drainage which prevents pooling and the feeling of leaden legs. Keep the body correctly aligned, with your weight equally on both feet. Feel long and elastic with the tension distributed evenly throughout your body. This will help prevent development of impacted muscles, particularly in the thighs.

You should be animated and exhilarated and far from exhaustion.

3 Use springs and kicks to relieve the pressure in the legs. Combine these with strong movements in the upper body, which act like a body pump, and work to push up your heart rate. Use your breathing as a guide to whether or not you are working at a reasonable level – it should be easy and not forced.

You will need fifteen to twenty minutes of fairly sustained work on your feet in order to gain the benefits of stamina work.

Remember that you are your own best timekeeper, so be sensible, don't overdo it and work only for as long as you feel comfortable.

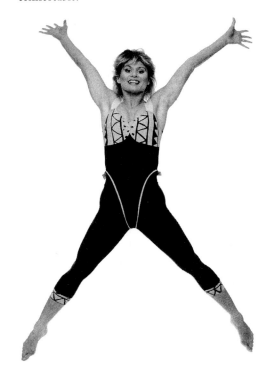

4 Do not stop moving completely even if you feel uncomfortable. Simply slow down and ease out your shoulders, keeping the steps going until you feel ready to take off again. To add variety, try different music and make up new step combinations, or put your track suit on and do your stamina programme outside from time to time, possibly increasing the running and jogging.

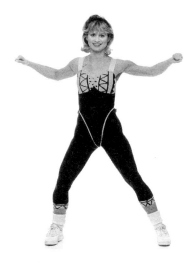

marching and stepping. You can use the Warm Up section from page 57 as a starting point to get you going.

Here are some simple routines to use as starting points:

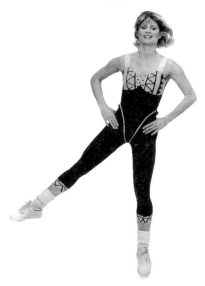

5 Vary the music. The main object is to keep going and avoid boredom. The body tends to resist the trauma of stamina work. You could say that 'your muscles can't hear the music'.

I always find that there are two main crash barriers to get through – the heat and sweat barrier and the deep breathing barrier. Steer safely through these and you will be away and running in top gear.

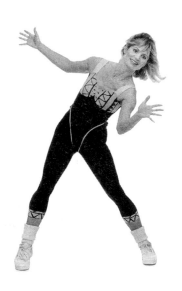

6 Try to get as much fresh air as possible. If you like to watch the time closely, try to reach the highest speed and intensity at between eight and twelve minutes. Use the last four to six minutes out of, say, twenty to slow down very gradually into

Try doing each movement to a count of 8 or 16 and be conscious of the rhythm.

1 Start with heel presses on the spot. Then lift the feet and take the movement into marching. Walk forwards and backwards with rhythm, then step sideways left and right, clapping your hands together after every fourth step.

2 Step-and-kick and step-and-kick, clapping your hands on each kick. Then walk on the spot for a count of 8 and then return to step-kicking. Now take the movement into jogging on the spot before taking it into jogging on the move. Return to step-kicking, then jog, then kick.

3 Try doing 'jumping jacks' (star jumps) and side steps: step-together-step-together. Then step and jump, raising alternate knees high and clapping your hands under each one.

Any variation on these can be used. Just make sure you keep up the pressure: marching, side-stepping, jogging, skipping, running, any

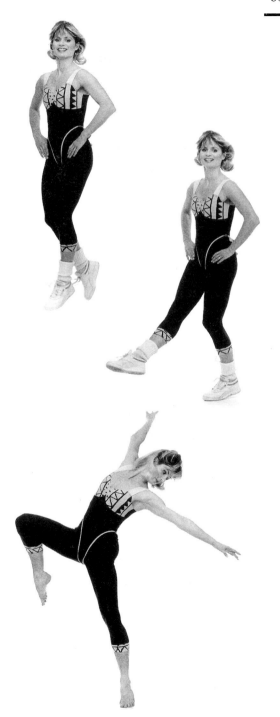

dance or disco step you might
know. Change the
direction you are facing.

Try at some point to get your
knees up to hip level, ease out your
shoulders and keep your neck free.
This is not the time to let your
body flop. You need to feel as
strongly resilient as a bouncing
rubber ball.

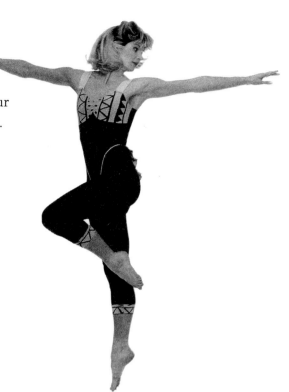

11   *Suppleness: the Energy of Air*

TIME: 15 MINUTES
MUSIC: SMOOTH, FLOWING, NOT TOO FAST

What do We Mean by Suppleness?

When we think about the subtle inter-play of tendons, ligaments, joints and muscles, we are thinking about suppleness. It is about realigning the body and releasing tension in the muscles. It will enable you to find new levels of energy to revitalize your life and will help you to bend and move with the ease you had as a child.

Because the joints need to be loaded to release the lubricating fluid, and the muscles and tendons need to be encouraged to stretch and lengthen, we always combine strong movements with easy flowing movements, creating the ideal situation for achieving both – this is the suppleness system – and it will help you to avoid the stiffness which sometimes follows vigorous exercise.

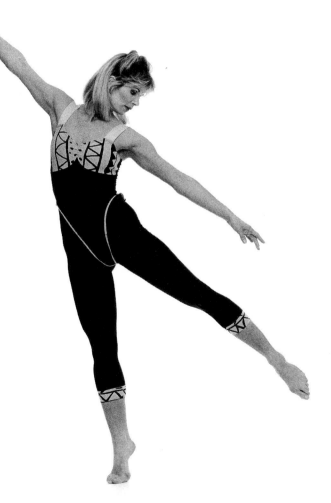

All conscious movement takes place across a joint. It is easy to understand the need to keep them healthy and mobile. Our quality of life is directly related to the ease with which we can move our joints!

Nothing is more immediately limiting than the loss of use of even one joint. If you have ever nursed a stiff knee or elbow for a single day, you will know what I mean.

Knowing the way a joint is made up can help you to understand its importance.

About the Joints

Joints hold the body in correct or incorrect alignment which relates directly to a permanently stressed or stress-free body. Joints are formed where two or more bones meet. They are the junction or connection between the hard, stable levers of bone, and set the style, shape and range of movement of the limbs or any part of the body.

There are several sorts of joint. These can be divided mainly into hinge, gliding, and ball and socket joints, and we learn unconsciously from infancy exactly how each joint works. Watch a baby kicking, and see how it uses its knees like hinges, but happily allows the legs to fall outwards, rotating from the ball and socket hip joint.

Each bone ends in a spongy layer of cartilage. This protects the head of the bone and the joint acting as a shock absorber, and also in childhood protecting the epiphyses, or growing points of the bone. The joint itself is contained within a delicate membrane (the synovial membrane) which, when the joint is under pressure, secretes a lubricating fluid, called synovial fluid. This allows the joints to move more smoothly, greatly reducing general wear and tear.

Around each joint, protecting and holding it in place, are the strong, tough, dense ligaments. These tough fibres attach bone to bone and form something like a protective capsule around the joint. The knee, for instance, has seven ligaments holding it in place. Ligaments, though not rigid, are non-elastic and promote stability and strength.

The tendons, which are the tough ends of the muscle bundles with their covering fascia, attach the muscle to the bone. They, with the muscle, are more elastic than the ligaments, and are kept in good condition through regular exercise, allowing for the maximum range of movement of the joint. Tendons, because they are elastic, tend to shorten when not in use.

We sometimes talk of the inner, middle and outer range of the joint. This means simply that small everyday movements involve the inner range; making a conscious effort to enlarge or increase the extent of these movements would involve the middle range; while only dancers, acrobats, or those needing to display or project a body shape, would use the outer range. We sometimes call this 'high flexibility', and it can be hazardous and more to do with art than fitness! Some bodies are naturally more supple than others – the joints are more shallow and the ligaments and tendons less tight. Everyone, however, needs to work at suppleness.

Preparing for Suppleness

It is most essential to be warm when you begin, so that the muscles are more pliable, your body system is working more efficiently, and you will feel motivated to begin stretching. If you are doing this section on its own make sure you repeat the five-minute Warm Up at the beginning of Part 1 or have a warm bath. Take off your shoes, but wear socks and leg warmers to keep feet and ankles warm.

Most of this section involves sitting or lying on the floor, so to make yourself comfortable work on a firm but springy surface. Carpets, gym mats or foam rubber surfaces are ideal, but do not use a bed! Try to feel easy and at home, using the floor to help relax and realign the body. In class I say, 'make friends with the floor'. The postural muscles come under strain as they keep you upright, and the discs in the back tend to become compressed during the day. It is, therefore, good to relieve the muscles by lying on the floor.

Have some cushions or pillows to prop up your back or head if you feel more comfortable like this. You will also find that an increase of muscle tone will protect the pressure points and the floor will not seem too firm. This should provide you with an added incentive to be conscientious about the Strength section!

The Movements

This section works through the joints in the middle range, starting at the top and working down the body, focusing on each joint. Never forget that the whole body is involved, and do not 'cut off' the part you are working on. I have given some indication of the number of repetitions for each exercise, but you should use that as a guideline only. It is important in this section to do as many as you feel you want or need to.

Neck

1   Keep the neck free by turning the head and lightly balancing it at the top of the spine. Open your mouth to release the jaw. Face front and press the head gently forwards. Raise and tilt the chin upwards to 45 degrees. As a guideline, look two thirds of the way up the wall. Turn your head sideways and to the front four times, then combine this with pressing the chin forwards and down. Incline your head to one side and up, then to the other side, also four times.

Move very slowly and firmly. Any combinations are possible, but do not roll the head across the back, which can damage the top of the spine.

This can be done sitting on an upright chair.

Shoulders (ball and socket)

2a Roll your shoulders alternately, four times on each side. Change the dynamic or weight of the movement, so that it is sometimes strong and sometimes light. Think of the arms as wings and involve the back as you rotate the joint.

2b Rotate both arms together, keeping the neck free, i.e. not jutting forward and clamped like a ship's figurehead. We tend to lean forward a great deal after all, our eyes look ahead, and it all happens out there in front! It is therefore a good idea to emphasize the backward direction in these movements to counter our habitual forward focus. Try to feel the back hanging from the shoulder girdle, like a coat on a hanger, rather than hunched up towards your ears.

Upper Back

3 Circle the arms, crossing them in front and emphasizing the top of the circle, to counter the pull of gravity. Involve the ribcage very strongly. Take your time and see if you can yawn as you lift the ribcage to increase the action of the diaphragm and to maximize oxygen intake.

Forward Flexion

4 Wriggle your shoulders and release the back leaning forwards with bent knees, pulling in the abdominals. Then arch your back and move upward to the vertical. Imagine you are stacking the spine like a string of cotton reels from the pelvis upwards into space. Feel the energy and strength through the whole back.

5 Here we are using the action of sitting on the floor as part of the exercise.

  Put one knee down to the floor, leaning forwards and arching and rounding the back, taking the weight of the upper body on the hands, which should be on the floor. Now slowly lean both knees down, easing out the lower back (see movement 23 on page 78), and change to sitting cross legged on the floor.

Arms

6 Sit up straight on the sitting bones, with your legs crossed, head well balanced and the upper back flat. Keep the arms outstretched and twist them from the shoulder, bringing your elbows, hands and fingers

into the movement. Sit on a cushion or have your knees up in front, if you are uncomfortable. Repeat slowly eight times.

Lateral Flexion

7 Stretch out sideways, sliding your hand along the floor, then come back to sitting upright, before stretching out to the other side. This is lateral flexion of the spine. You should feel the stretch in the ribcage. Repeat four times on each side.

Lumbar/Lower Back

8a Now very slowly tilt forward from the pelvis, keeping the back straight and the abdominals pulled in firmly. You can keep your legs crossed as you do this or, if you prefer, straighten them out slightly, but make sure you keep the knees bent.

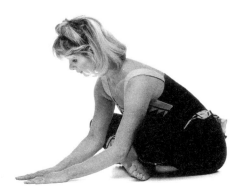

Push the knees down and feel the long, strong pull forwards from the lumbar spine. Really savour this, tilting the pelvis and relieving the intense pressure that is suffered by the lower back. The lower back is particularly prone to pressure as it not only supports the main body weight, but is also attached to the sacrum, which is fixed and, therefore, inflexible.

8b Now very slowly and carefully raise the arms as you come back to sitting upright, and twist the upper body towards the wall behind you, following each twist with the forward tilt. The movement should go like this – push forward, come up, then twist and come back, forward and up, then alternate the side twist. Take the head round sometimes, or keep facing front. Carry the body weight high and out of the hips to relieve pressure in the lower back.

You may hold any part of the movement if you wish, pressing firmly, but never flopping.

Feet and Knees

9a Ease out the legs, straightening them in front, propping yourself up on your hands, which should be behind you. This helps to keep the back straight.

9b Rotate the feet, pointing the toes, then push down the heels. Bend and straighten the knees alternately, moving lightly. The knees are usually under great pressure carrying the body weight. It is good to move them lightly, carefully feeling the possibility of extending the movement. Put a cushion behind you if you find it helps.

Lower Back

10a Keeping the hands behind you, bend the elbows slightly, pulling in the abdominals and pushing the hollow back towards the floor. You are reversing the hollow of your back. Raise the knees, keeping them hip width apart to assist the back, then lift the feet off the floor, leaning right back on the elbows. Your shin bones should be parallel with the floor. Feel balanced and comfortable.

10b Breathe deeply and do not tilt the head backwards but keep the chin tucked in.

Now take this into a rocking movement by alternately rocking forward and then back. Rock gently from side to side, focusing the body weight in the small of the back. This is a very small movement. This is a most refreshing, revitalizing position and a great aid to curing the pain so often associated with the overworked lower back. Prop yourself up on cushions if you feel the neck and shoulders are strained.

Hips

11a Keeping your arms wide apart on the floor behind you, push up into sitting with the feet apart and legs straight. Twist and press one hip forward to

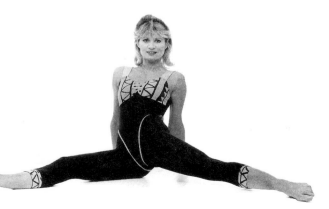

flatten the groin, releasing the other leg. Roll across, pulling in the abdominals and pressing out the hollow back and twist to the opposite side. Move slowly and hold the position.

11b Bend the front knee so as to increase the stretch in the groin, and hold. It is very common for women especially, because of heels and hollow backs, never quite to straighten out the groin. This leads to incorrect alignment and a pelvis which is permanently tipped forward. Move slowly and persuade your body to relax into the floor and give the muscles time to stretch. Repeat on the other side.

12a Straighten both legs and, keeping the back firm, lean forwards, reaching out towards

your feet. Try to keep your knees as straight as possible, and the chest up, and pull out the back of the legs. Hold for an increasing length of time, starting with a count of ten.

12b Move the arm across diagonally to increase the intensity of the stretch. Make sure you keep breathing rhythmically!

Spine

13a Roll backwards, flattening the spine piece by piece – remember the cotton reels! Stretch out the arms and legs into the St Andrew's Cross, flattening the palms of your hands, with the thumbs facing downwards, and making as much of the back as possible touch the floor. Feel the energy from the earth, and imagine two tracks crossing through the body from opposite hands and feet. Hold the position, pressing the heels down, and breathe deeply.

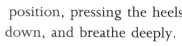

13b Curl up to cap the knees with the hands, crossing the feet and rounding the back. Rock gently and, keeping the abdominals pulled up, push the middle back towards the floor.

14 Gently lower the head to the floor and, still holding the knees lightly with feet crossed, rock gently from side to side and forwards and back.
Take your time, massaging the lower back into the floor. It can help to place a cushion under the pelvis. Try to feel that the spine is being lengthened downwards, like pulling a fox by the tail.

15 Stretch out slowly with arms kept at shoulder level on the floor, bend one knee and press it across the thigh. Feel the twist and stretch down the side then press the knee down flat on the other side, opening the hip joint.

16 Press both knees across and down, using the weight of the legs to hang into the floor. Keep the shoulders flat and turn your head away from the knees to increase the twist. Breathe freely and try not to overarch the hollow back. Flatten and ease out your back as you move the knees across, even lifting the feet if it helps. Allow one knee to sink down to the floor, guiding it with your hand. Open the pelvis and allow the other knee to follow across.
Hold and pause on any part of the movement you wish. Try to feel inwardly and let go as much as possible. Try to melt into the floor.

Legs

17 The legs are under constant pressure from the weight of the body, impeding circulation and fluid (lymphatic) drainage. That 'My legs feel like lead'

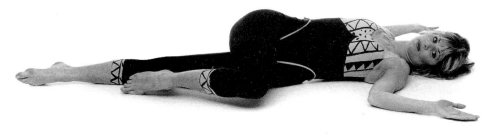

feeling really can have a
physiological cause and it is
always good to get the feet up
to assist drainage back towards
the heart.

18 From a prone position, leaning
one leg on the floor and
propped up on
pillows if you need,
stretch the other leg upwards,
grasping below the knee. Aim
to straighten the knee if
possible. Hold as long as is
comfortable. Try not to strain
the neck and shoulders and
keep the abdominals pulled up.

19 Lift both legs together and
grasp the toes if possible – it
depends very much on how
long your arms are – or hold
below the knees. Imagine
the feet empty-
ing. Feel a strong
stretch down the back
of the legs. Remember
to keep breathing.

20 Allow the feet to sink outwards
using the weight of the legs to
pull the feet apart. Hold on to
the inner thighs if you are un-
happy with holding your feet.
Try to keep the legs straight,
but do not lock the knees.
Breathe into the stretch and
hold for as long as possible.

Do not feel desperate; these
stretches are hard work and
need to be held for at least a
count of twenty.

21a Lying on the floor, bend your
knees and slide your feet
together along the floor, with
your arms up above your head,
and do your own 'waking up
in the morning' stretch.

21b Slowly curl over to one side,
rounding the back, with the
elbows tucked in – this is the
foetal position – and sense
the security and strength of
the earth. Support your head

on an arm if you like.

Unroll and stretch out again, then very, very slowly curl up on the opposite side. Be easy with the way you feel, but do not flop. Feel relaxed but in control. This is not sleep time and you need to start thinking about getting up.

22 When you are ready, roll up on to your knees, still in the foetal position. Rest your head on your hands and allow your pelvis to sink back on your heels. Feel the long slow stretch through the back. If your knees protest, or you dislike having your head down, roll out on to your back, push yourself into a sitting position, then on to one knee and up (rather as you got down). Move the weight forward on to the hands, put one knee up and very slowly uncurling like a cat, come up into standing. (Refer back to the starting position on page 63.)

Give yourself time as changing the level of the body can alter the blood pressure and you could feel giddy.

Shake out the shoulders,

yawn, turn your head and balance your body weight between your feet by moving from one foot to the other. You should feel good – unstressed, correctly aligned, and stretched.

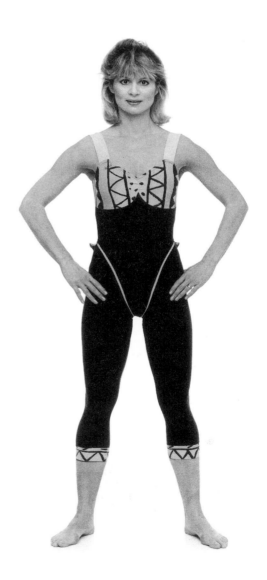

12 *Wind Down*

TIME: 5 MINUTES
MUSIC: VERY SLOW, STRONG

Why We Need Harmony and Inner Calm

This last section of the workout can be experienced on many levels. It can be done as a simple section of calming, balancing and strengthening movements, or it may be felt on a deeper level as something nearer to a meditation in movement, emptying the mind of anxiety and the body of stress.

Approach it in a way that is right for *you*, and always trust your intuition about what is right for you on any particular day.

The sequence of movements can be repeated as often as you wish; feel free to use it as a starting point for your own creative ideas on how to calm and harmonize your mind and body. Take it at your own pace and refuse to be interrupted! A calm mind affects the body, and a calm body affects the mind. Stress in either is a cause of fatigue and wasted energy.

The Movements

1 Stand with your feet comfortably apart, correctly balanced, and feel as if the spine extends upwards through the crown of your head. Imagine you are hanging in space, and release the tension in the neck by opening your mouth and slowly turning your head from one side to the other.

2 Slow down your breathing, starting with a controlled out breath. Concentrate on the turning point of your breathing, which is when breathing out becomes breathing in.

3 Try to look inwards and be aware of your own space. Be aware of your body shape and think outwards, fixing this shape into the space around you. Balance your awareness of both spaces, your inner space and the outer space, feel at ease with both. Try to detach yourself for a moment, accept this person — yourself — as she is. Feel respect and kindness towards her. Give yourself time to feel serene and confident in stillness.

4 Now feel the pulse and vitality of life in your body, marvel at your strength and feel the energy of the earth through your feet, carrying your body upwards into space.

5 When you begin, move with great concentration and inner intensity, allowing one movement to flow smoothly into the next.

  Raise your arms out in an arc from your sides until they are stretched up above your head. Then pull your arms down strongly in front of your body, bending your elbows towards the pelvis, rounding the back, bending the knees and pulling in the abdominal muscles.

6 Breathe in as you go down, then out as your arms go up. Reverse the breathing and repeat each cycle four times, or as often as you wish. Be aware of your strength and grow out of the ground. End with your arms high.

7 From the high vertical stretch lower your arms alternately down to the sides and back in a

wide arc, tracing a circle in the air, leaving one arm pinned in the air, and exploring the space with the other. Do not flop at any time, but feel strong and calm. Be intuitive about what feels right for you, altering the pace and frequency of the stretches as you wish.

8   Bring both arms down to shoulder level and raise one knee. Breathe deeply and feel your body weight balanced on one leg. Use any shape for balance which is comfortable, but requires an effort of quiet concentration.

9   Without actually touching, run your hands down your sides, 'shaping' your body down to your ankles and then up to cross over your head. Feel the life and energy radiating from your body and the warmth and strength in your hands as they cross over your head. This should be a blessing, an act of loving. Think of the space your body occupies and claim it – it is for you alone.

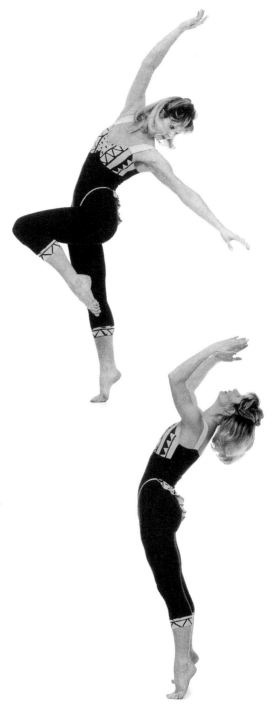

10 Use the energy lines to stretch out and balance the body (see page 74). Feel the energy and life force from fingertips to toes crossing through the body from earth into space and back again.

Without jarring, swing your hands strongly downwards to cross in front, contracting the body inwards. Using the strength and energy of the pelvis, push up and hold the body in extension on the energy line positions in any sequence you like. Feel full of calm control and, if it comes naturally, balance on the balls of your feet by pushing your weight forward slightly.

11 Do your posture check, as in the Warm Up, aligning your head, shoulders and hips, and bring the arms down to the sides. Yawn, smile and open and close your eyes.

Look outwards calmly and face the day.

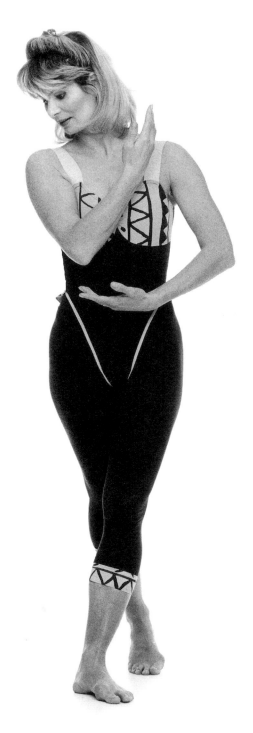

If you have worked through the whole programme you should feel warm, glowing and invigorated, not exhausted. Even without the intensity of the work in the Strength or Stamina sections, you need to move with enough inner concentration to achieve this glow. Never flop or move in 'neutral' which is, for the most part, the way we move in daily life. It may be economical of effort but it is not useful as a training exercise. Always keep the strong, smooth current of movement, rather like the quality of Tai Chi, which warms and strengthens the body and avoids completely the discomfort and wear and tear of jolting the body through stopping and starting.

If you are working with the video and have learned the patterns of movement and know how the body should feel, you can be more creative and introduce some ideas of your own, especially in the Warm Up and Stamina sections.

The programme should be a springboard, a starting point only, and you should never allow yourself to feel stale. Dead repetitive exercise is no use to mind or body, and does more harm than good.

Keep a sense of wonder and intense inner pleasure in what you are doing, for each movement is unique and new, and is in itself a miracle.

Adapting Medau

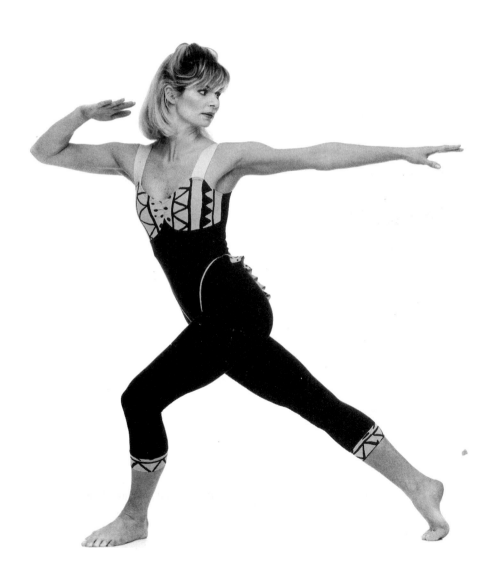

Medau is easily adapted to any age group because correct movement is everyone's natural starting point. Whether you are young or old, pregnant or with children, fit or want to be fitter, the following sections will show just how versatile and fun Medau is for everyone.

—

13 *Medau for the Under 5s*

Children take to Medau instinctively. After all, it is the child's natural way of moving: easy; unaffected; right for their bodies; expressing their personalities and mood of the moment.

Hinrich Medau constantly reminded his students to study children at play. Recapturing their suppleness and energy became one of the cornerstones of his teaching.

All young creatures unconsciously learn through movement. This is not just fitness and physical skills, but how to behave, interrelate and understand how the world works. They need endless time to experiment and a safe place to explore. They need a kindly, unflustered adult, a peer group, and days of playing and 'pottering' in a wonderful round of animation and sleep.

Sadly today, there is neither time nor space for this idyllic scheme and children's lives are often as complex and crowded as their parents. Strapped for hours in car seats and buggies, 'parked' in front of the television, reduced to a temper in hot, crowded supermarkets, the modern child has little time for this vital, natural play.

With such busy lives few children have enough free time to themselves. They love and need to move; it helps them to become confident, fit and strong.

Most parents understand that children are in a constant state of flux, developing and changing at high speed. You need to be one jump ahead and anticipate the basic developmental patterns which emerge with the growing child. The bold, assertive four year old, kicking a football with a will to win, is not the same as the cooperative three year old who, a year ago, delighted in threading beads and singing rhymes.

Their interests focus on different areas as they grow. They are not mini-adults. Imagine how confusing it would be to have a complete change of body shape and personality every few months. Children need time to get to grips with themselves. By setting the pace for themselves, discovering their own inner rhythm and way of doing things – without feeling that they have got it all wrong – children develop into happy, healthy human beings.

Lala and I have devised a method of working with children which uses their natural play patterns and gives them plenty of scope for their own variations. This should never be regimented, but designed to suit the age group and to use a child's instinctive response to movement and rhythm. The children are allowed to achieve and develop at their own pace.

Medau's work with props has been an invaluable source of ideas. For instance, the large soft balls are used in many ways: for skill and agility in throwing and chasing; for strength in squeezing; for balance in perching on them; and for socializing in swapping and rolling them away.

The classes are full of fun, music and rhythm, but always have a clear structure of movement and fitness themes, as well as aiming to use the whole space of the room imaginatively. The following points are adhered to closely:

- Strength and skill using their sense of adventure.
- Music and rhythm in group work.
- Fine movements involving hand/eye coordination.
- Fantasy, mime, dancing can all play a part. There has to be a special atmosphere of free enterprise, generosity and basic good manners.

The release and happiness that can be seen when working with children underlines the need for them to have time and a safe place to be themselves.

'Class' at Home

It can be great fun to clear a space, put on some music, take off your shoes and dance together. Children respond instinctively to rhythm and music and have a touching delight in moving in a group or with an adult. Call it your class if you like.

Warm Up

Skip, jump and 'bop', moving freely around the room, changing directions, exploring the corners, running into the centre, crossing over . . . you will get plenty of instructions from the over 2s on how you should dance. Babies love to be carried and rocked to the music.

Stretch

Now do some stretches. Reach for the sky. How far up the wall can you touch?

Lie down on the floor and stretch out like a star – catch your feet, keeping your knees straight. Gently stretch small arms, legs, feet and hands.

Most children love being turned upside-down to hang from knees or ankles. This aligns and stretches the spine.

Strength and Coordination

Children love tricks. They will suddenly discover that they can spin round and round and will practise endlessly. Try things out together, starting on the floor.

Roll backwards with your feet in the air. Roll over and over. Wriggle on your tummy, crawl, do head over heels, 'swim' on your front. The variations are endless and delightful.

When my children were small we used to turn the room into a large 'track', clambering over the sofa, under the table, rolling over the rug, jumping up from the chair then running to start again! This sort of play develops strength and coordination. Learning to balance and manage weight is the first step towards becoming a safe child.

Singing

It is a joy to sing and act rhymes together. All the old-fashioned ones: 'Humpty-Dumpty', 'Ring-o-Roses', 'Miss Muffet' still charm, and there are plenty of new ones. You must both do it. The fun disappears if you spend 10 minutes on the telephone, refusing to be interrupted. Many small children, especially the 2-4s, love fantasy and mime:

'I'm a rabbit/big bad wolf. . .'
'I'm making a cake/driving the car, etc'

These are excellent starting points for even more ambitious games.

Fun for Toddlers

Coordination

Try this with a small child, aged
betweeen 2-5 years, but bear in
mind that it might need adapting
to the particular age and tempera-
ment of the child.

ACTION	PURPOSE
Find two brown paper bags.	
Put one on your hand and wave to me.	*Social contact*
Now your left/right hand.	*Are they following?*
Wave up high – now to the side – now behind you.	*Concept of directions*
Can you put it on your foot like a shoe? Have mine – that makes two shoes.	*Counting and fantasy*
Be careful not to tear it.	
Let's fold it across like this, and see if you can make it flutter like a bird.	*Hand/eye coordination*
Run about with it – is it a bird flying or a fish wiggling?	*Stamina*
Let it float down like a dry leaf – catch it before it lands.	*Skill and agility*
Balance on it.	*Balance*

There are endless variations:

Make a hole and peep through
(2 years)

Make a hat (3 years)

Draw a face and make a hand
puppet (4–5 years)

Scrunch it up and make a ball
(4–5 years)

Blow it up and bang it (4–5 years).

Expensive toys are not needed
when children can produce exciting
ideas with almost anything. There
should be a special atmosphere of
give and take between the child and
the adult, as well as respect for each
other's space. Children spend so
much time on the receiving end of
an adult's attention with little time
to contribute anything themselves;
this is their chance.

Their pace and energy patterns
are quite different from an adult's.
They rush about, they flop, take
forever over some things; their
interest span seems minimal and
they have a trick of doing the
opposite to what is expected.
Always try to give them time to
move freely and to organize
themselves at their own pace. Apply
everything you do in class to all
their other activities: balance on the
garden wall; skip to the post box
and sing in the car.

Many childhood problems are
eased through the release and joy
that free movement brings. Basic
learning concepts are unconsciously
absorbed – judging height, weight,
distance, shape, direction, numbers,
using and understanding words,
memory training and creativity.

Childhood is not totally about
advanced learning concepts or even
laying down sensible fitness habits
for a lifetime. Remember always
that in childhood mind and body
are one, and in moving together
you are dealing with profundities.

14　*Medau for the Over 40s*

I never minded reaching forty. My body seemed stronger and in many ways more stable. There seemed to be fewer swings of energy and mood, less wavering about decisions, more economy of effort and a greater general competence about life. The children were less demanding on a day-to-day basis and time seemed to expand a little. So feel positive and use the manifold advantages of reaching this age.

The Art of Energy needs little or no adaptation for the over 40s, but for the less fit here are some helpful suggestions:

1　Be intuitive about how you feel and what seems right for you. There is a fine line between overtaxing and underachieving. You must have a clear picture of how fit you want to be and be realistic about your goals. Aim to build up your strength and stamina gradually, but keep the pressure up.

2　All the floor work can be done quite simply with the help of a cushion placed strategically under the head or buttocks. Experiment and see what helps most to make the movement easier.

3　Avoid the deep knee bend (pliés) – do the same movement but with a more shallow bend if the knees feel strained.

4　'Cheat' happily in the Strength section. You do not want to use only your large 'emergency' muscles, but persuade your body to use the unfamiliar ones too. Push up with support from the arms to help when tightening the abdominals. Never load the joints to the point of discomfort. Keep the neck free from strain by constantly easing out.

5 Take a little more time to get up and down when doing floor work. This movement alters the blood pressure and you might feel giddy.

6 If the floor seems miles away, most of the floor work can be done in a chair. Feel free to experiment.

7 Change the pace of the strong movements to 'half time' if it seems more suitable. For example, the leg lifts to tighten the buttocks: do them slowly and rest frequently.

8 Be sensible about the Stamina section. Be careful of your feet and do not distress your body. Walk rather than jog, or skip, if it is easier. It helps to use the room space so that you can try your own variations. At the end, you should feel exhilarated but not exhausted.

9 Be conscientious about the Suppleness section. Joints tend to stiffen from now on and need to be moved regularly.

10 Check your posture carefully as shown in the programme. The pull of gravity begins to take its toll and an increasing effort has to be made to defeat it.

11 Pander a little more to your mood and energy level. The body may not be less willing but it certainly grows more cunning at avoiding effort. Persuade, cajole and give yourself time to get your breathing going before launching into the whole programme.

Medau makes you look and feel good, preserving a youthful elasticity in the muscles.

15 *Medau for the Over 60s*

This age group includes me. I am prejudiced of course, but I think that Medau is superb for older people. With correct, natural movement you never have the depressing feeling that things are falling apart.

Your fitness movement programme simply adapts to suit you. It looks good and feels right and if high stamina does not appeal at the moment, then try stretching, keeping the joints supple, strengthening the muscles and doing some breathing.

Most of the Art of Energy is perfectly suitable if performed at a much slower pace. Do not rush, and take what you need from the programme. Try to do some exercise every day – as even one day missed seems to make starting again a little harder. Be easy and relaxed about it and take time to get into the swing of things.

Keeping the joints mobile is the first priority: stretching and contracting the muscles, wriggling and yawning can be an on-going daily occupation.

Classes for older people can be full of rhythmic music and the creative use of hand apparatus (props such as cushions). The variety and ease of movement makes Medau ideal for this age group.

Here is a workout which can be done simply, sitting in a chair:

Warm Up
Sit comfortably in a stout, upright chair. Rub your hands, face, elbows and knees. Now warm and rub your arms and thighs.

Put on your favourite dance music. Still sitting, rock, hop, clap, sing, stamp your feet and enjoy the rhythm with many variations. Be as energetic and creative or easy as you like, but feel warm and glowing at the end.

Stretches

Sit up straight with your feet and knees hip width apart, pressing the lower back against the chair. Balance your head, opening your mouth, turning gently to left and right. Feel as if you are hanging from the ceiling through the crown of your head. Stretch out your arms in any direction you fancy, feeling the stretch run through from one set of fingertips to the other.

Holding the sides of the chair, stretch your legs and feet out in front of you and bend and stretch each leg alternately — about eight times.

Suppleness

This will ease the joints. Choose slow, soft music. Very carefully, starting with releasing the jaw, go right through the body, moving every joint you can find. Enjoy it — marvel at how your fingers, elbows, shoulders work. Lightly holding the sides of the chair and keeping the back extended, rock forwards and back (eight times) then from side to side (eight times).

Strength

Squeeze a cushion with your hands (count to eight). Hug it. Press it against your chest and then abdomen (counting to eight each time). Squeeze it between your knees (count to eight). Hold it in your hands like a tray and lift carefully to nose level (count to four). Toss the cushion away, get up carefully and move around the room, gently swaying and responding to the music. Open a window and breathe freely. Practise balancing on one leg while holding on to the chair. You should feel wonderful.

Never stop moving. Play your favourite music and feel exhilarated by the rhythm. Be respectful of your body. It is an old friend. Be constantly safety conscious — avoiding careless accidents which take time and energy to overcome.

Be aware of your general health and be sensible about resting enough. Fatigue can sometimes be caused by boredom.

Movement will help to keep you strong, mobile, looking and feeling good. It is a source of infinite and increasing pleasure — whatever your age.

16   *Medau Through Your Pregnancy*

Proof that Medau produces a body that works for you is nowhere more evident than when you have a baby.

- It gives you a high level of general fitness (see Health Benefits, page 31).

- The emphasis on correct body alignment helps you to avoid lower back pain and other common postural problems.

- Your muscles will be long, strong and elastic – not heavy and bulky – which means that the extra weight you carry in pregnancy is more easily accommodated and your post-natal recovery will be much quicker: the muscles will spring back more quickly.

- Good breathing technique and a calm mind are a great help during the birth itself.

Medau helps you towards an increased awareness and respect for your body, so that you keep in touch with the changes which happen so quickly. However well prepared you are, the experience of pregnancy and childbirth is highly individual and Medau's intuitive approach will help you to accept and understand the whole process with greater ease.

Provided, always, that there are no complications in the first three months it is perfectly safe to use the Art of Energy video workout for as long as it feels comfortable. With some adjustments, you can have fun and benefit from rhythmic movement up to delivery day.

How to Adapt the Art Of Energy

During the first three months, be intuitive about your energy levels.

The changes in your body can make you feel nauseous and exhausted. Give yourself time to settle in: put on the Art of Energy video and 'pretend' to be exercising; enjoy watching Lala do the work! You will be learning the patterns, relaxing with the rhythm and unconsciously picking up excellent tips about good posture and general body management.

1 Stretch: the Energy of Water

During pregnancy the body produces a hormone called relaxin. This helps to relax the joints, especially in the pelvis, in preparation for the birth. Do not overstretch or become too flexible even if you feel more than usually supple. Joints can become unstable and so it is vital that the back, knees and hips, especially, are kept in correct alignment.

Avoid the deep knee bends – do only a slight or half bend instead. Remember that your back will be coping without the help of your abdominal muscles, so do only half twists. Check your posture and do pelvic tilts to ease out the lower back.

Always have plenty of cushions handy when doing the floor exercises: as your tummy grows you will need them to support your back. If you find the floor uncomfortable, try sitting in a chair. The weight of the baby pressing on the large blood vessels in the pelvis can make you feel faint, so the cushions will help.

Later, your abdominal muscles will not be able to support the spine: they will be too stretched to contract and so you may have to abandon some of these exercises. Do not worry – the muscles will shrink back in their own time after the birth – even before you begin exercising again.

Slow down the rhythm to half pace to accommodate your changing shape and increased weight. This means the repetitions of any movement will decrease in number.

Ease out your neck and shoulders constantly: the increased weight of your bust puts an added strain on the upper back.

2 Strength: the Energy of the Earth

Reduce the intensity of the work by more than half. While you need to exercise your muscles you must avoid pushing up your blood pressure. Try not to lift your body weight, but go halfway and have the sensation of lifting: this will contract and tone your muscles without straining your neck and back. Reach around only halfway with the body twists.

3 Stamina: the Energy of Fire

This can be moderated to suit your gradually changing needs. Walk rather than jog or skip and slow down whenever you please. Keep the windows open so you breathe lots of fresh air; drink when you are thirsty. Try not to get too hot: as much blood as possible is needed by the baby, so do not waste it by making it feed the large muscle groups as you leap about.

If your back and legs feel tired sit on a straight-backed chair and bop away. Enjoy the increased pace and rhythm. You will feel good and well exercised without having overtaxed your joints.

Watch out for your feet. Raise them higher than your pelvis whenever you can. Stretch and rotate the feet constantly to stimulate circulation and lymphatic drainage. This helps to reduce cramp in the legs and puffy ankles.

As you feel more earthbound try to think of carrying your body weight up as high as possible, concentrating on lightness and focusing upwards.

4 Suppleness: the Energy of Air

This is a lovely section for pregnancy – but be wary of becoming too supple. (See Stretch, page 113: the hips and knees, which take the main body weight, need to be very stable and must not swing about.)

Sit on a chair if you feel it will help to keep the back stable. Use the cushions to prop you up and only twist very gently and halfway.

Practise your breathing and balancing, using a wall or a heavy chair to keep you steady. Your centre of gravity will have altered which can make you wobble more than usual. Take more time to breathe: sometimes the diaphragm is pressed upwards and is unable to contract downwards so easily.

You will find that pregnancy has made you more aware of your body. Be sensitive and loving towards yourself and the growing baby inside you.

The Birth

Nothing that you read, or have learned from your ante-natal class, quite matches up with what happens on the day. Be very open-minded and follow the Medau rule of doing what feels right at the time. Birth is like a dance in three parts: you need to recognize the patterns and get swept up in the rhythm.

STAGE 1

Stay on your feet for as long as possible. Take in your favourite tapes and dance about. At this stage the uterus is contracting upwards, almost as if it is shrugging its shoulders to dilate the cervix. Support your back by leaning over the bed or pressing against the wall so that the strong contractions roll through your body. Move about between contractions: you need the force of gravity to help the baby along.

Some hospitals have a rocking chair to help when the contractions become more frequent. You can sit on an ordinary chair, knees apart, and rock forwards and backwards with a straight back (pelvic tilt). This eases out the lower back, relieves cramp and is thought to release – through the strong rhythmic movement – endorphins, the body's natural pain relievers.

STAGE 2

Once the baby's head is in the birth canal there is a compulsion to push downwards. Medau's emphasis on using the whole body means that every muscle group swings into action: this disperses the pressure evenly while the power and strength of the whole body concentrate in complete harmony.

Try to keep active – do not lie on your back like a beached whale gasping for breath. Rock on your hands and knees, sit up and squat with your knees bent up in front, holding on to one bent knee and then another. Keep in mind exactly what is happening and try to follow the dance.

Breathe up high in your lungs and pant if you are asked to slow down, always relaxing away from the contractions. Wait for the magic words, 'Push now'. The relief is exquisite. Be joyful: if you are lucky, giving birth can be superb.

The Post-Natal Period

Like spring time, the post-natal period can be less sunny and more exhausting than you anticipated.

Do not be impatient to regain your long-lost waistline: your body needs time to settle and in any case all your energy will be spent looking after the baby – broken nights can exhaust you completely.

Health is more important than fitness at this time and with the joints still loose, the pelvic floor overstretched and the back overworked, the rule must be later rather than sooner. You will be very vulnerable to long-term stress injuries: more harm can be done by unsuitable post-natal exercise than in all the nine months of pregnancy.

Be guided at the post-natal classes or by the hospital physiotherapist who will show you how to do pelvic floor contractions and encourage you to keep your legs moving to help stimulate your circulation. You can do some gentle pulling in by hugging your pillows and curling round them and then stretching out gently.

Do not worry about your shape. Believe that your body is doing its best for you. Do not increase your exhaustion at this crucial time: wait for the moment when you feel you need and want to exercise.

Follow the Art of Energy in the way you adapted it for your ante-natal programme. Be gentle with your abdominal muscles: if you struggle too hard then the back muscles will take over so that they are overstrained while the abdominals miss out altogether.

Be careful not to miss the perform-ance of pregnancy – it is such a tiny part of your life but it can have great intensity. Ride out the tears and tiredness: you will have touched life at its very beginnings and for many mothers this is more precious than all the rest.

17 *Whole Body Harmony*

Does Medau have a spiritual element? It certainly does not have to and works very well as a purely physical discipline. It depends on the sort of person you are, and on what you are looking for.

For some people, and for only some of the time, Medau can be a deeply satisfying, releasing experience, which can have an almost spiritual dimension. The excitement of the rhythm and the pleasure of discovering something 'right' and manageable for your body can be strangely uplifting.

I remember someone moved to tears after class, saying, 'All my life I've felt such a clumsy lump, but today I suddenly thought "My God – I'm dancing."' This was the beginning of a new confidence in herself and ultimate acceptance of much unhappiness in her childhood.

I have seen too many people thrilled and delighted to deny the fact that Medau can work on many levels of awareness. It is, however, a physical discipline, and I have little patience with romantic notions that do not at least begin with the aim of a well-trained body.

I am often asked what I, personally, feel about it. As a teacher my first task is to produce a useful class for the people in front of me. But, in truth, that is only half of the story. I have a profound respect for the work and the joy it brings. It is sometimes like being in touch with the vast life force, and seeing this energy awakened in others can seem magical.

Perhaps, through movement, we do sometimes capture that strange rhythmical pulse which we might call 'life'.

I am not sure, but I do know that I never finish class without feeling that through all the noise and 'romping', there has been a sharing of something rare and sweet and elemental. Who knows if we can call that 'spiritual'?

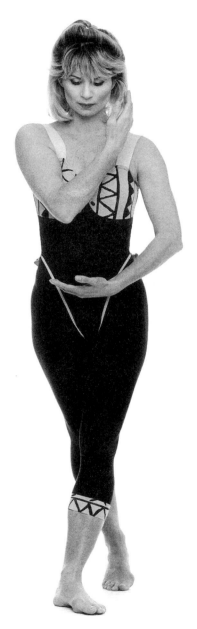

Professional Tributes

Lucy has been one of my dearest friends since we met on her first visit to the Medau school.

She was in her early twenties, and I remember her vividly then and see her still as 'one of the bright and the beautiful'.

Her grasp of Medau's work was immediate and instinctive. Her supreme gifts as a teacher (I count myself amongst her admiring pupils) and her long experience make anything she does authentic and authoritative.

It is a joy to see Lala developing the work through the modern media with an elegance and ease which would have delighted Medau himself.

I send them every blessing and wish every success to this important book and video *Medau: the Art of Energy*.

I look forward to more creations from this glowing partnership which has already contributed so much to the unfolding development of our beloved Medau.

Peggy Secord, President of the Medau Society and the person who brought Medau to Britain

Medau: the Art of Energy combines the best on offer for both fitness and movement. The whole body is exercised rhythmically with one movement flowing naturally into the next. It preserves the best of Medau's long experience with a completely contemporary approach. It is great fun to do and absolutely right for people in the 90s.

Elaine Burgess
The Sports Council

The enthusiasm and energy of Lucy Jackson shine through her teaching of whole body movement as illustrated in this interesting and important book. She expresses her justifiable belief in the safe graduated programme of movement which balances mind and body. She makes Medau accessible to everyone and the illustrations and video are beautifully presented by Lala Manners who, like her mother, is a stunning tribute to the efficacy of Medau.

Sir George Pinker KCVO
Harley Street

The Medau College runs many international courses for students of PE, dance or medicine during vacations. Schloss Hohenfels is still the nerve centre of the Medau world and a place to which all Medau teachers return with a sense of homecoming.

Medau Schule
Schloss Hohenfels
Coburg
Germany

The Medau Society in the UK:
8b Robson House
East Street
Epsom
Surrey KT17 1HH

Lucy Jackson can be contacted at:
23 Springfield Road
London NW8 0QJ

Lucy Jackson BA Hons (London), doyenne of Medau in Britain, has taught fitness, movement and dance classes for almost forty years. Her enthusiasm and expertise have made her the most famous exponent of the Medau Method. She has taken the work all over the world and is the author of countless articles on Medau and health-related topics. Married to gynaecologist Ian Jackson, she has a daughter, Lala Manners, and twin sons.

Lala Manners BA Hons Dip Ed (London), Lucy's daughter, was born to the Medau Method and shares her mother's passion for movement. She has studied all fields of movement, dance and exercise, and teaches extensively. Renowned for her work with babies and children, she is becoming increasingly well-known for her appearances on television and throughout the media.

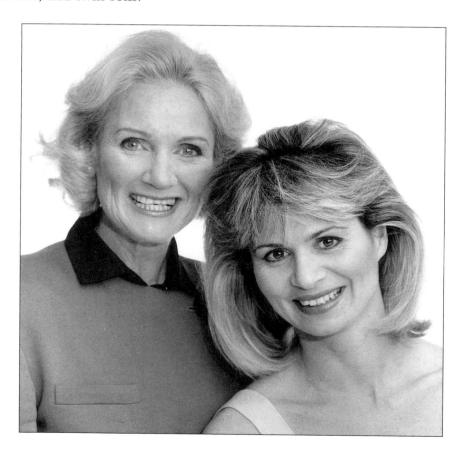

Medau

THE ART OF ENERGY

—

The Polygram Video

The bestselling video *Medau: The Art of Energy* is produced by Polygram and features Lala Manners who presents the video.

The video is available from W H Smith, Woolworths and all good video stores and is priced from £10.99.

"Medau is the exercise movement for every woman, whatever your age or fitness level – it's fun, graceful and balanced, teaching whole-body movements, suppleness and rhythm."

GOOD HOUSEKEEPING

"For those of us who are always intending to start exercising – soon – MEDAU could be just the incentive!"

WOMAN'S WEEKLY

"MEDAU has been around for a very long time and is likely to be here for a long time to come."

MARIE CLAIRE

"With MEDAU there is no gain through pain – movement flows through the body putting no stress to the joints. The aim is to strengthen and harmonise mind and body rather than exhaust them."

WOMAN'S REALM

"MEDAU stretches the body in the most natural way."

VOGUE

Bodyfit

Josh Salzmann

'Training with Josh is always fun'
JOHN CLEESE (*A FISH CALLED WANDA*)

Josh Salzmann is a one to one Personal Fitness Trainer.

He knows we're all different – and his programme will help you discover just what is right for you!

Josh Salzmann's *Bodyfit* will give you energy for life!

Josh Salzmann's revolutionary approach to fitness is simple, fun and safe to do. His exercises can be done Anywhere, Anytime, by Anyone!

Whether at home, at work, on holiday or on business, follow the *Bodyfit* programme just 3 times a week and discover how easy it is to add fitness to your lifestyle.

- Learn how to plan your Personal Fitness Programme
- Add fun and variety to your daily routine with Josh's *extra* exercises
- Enjoy a workout with your partner
- Exercise *safely* in the gym
- Discover your new route to *complete* health and fitness and start to change your life *right now!*

0 7225 2691 1   £7.99

The Natural Beauty Book

Cruelty free cosmetics to make at home

Anita Guyton

Have you ever stopped to consider what you
are putting on your face?

- Most shop-bought cosmetics are unpleasant mixtures of
chemicals and dead matter, have been tested on animals
and contribute to the destruction of our environment.

- There is an alternative – it will benefit your skin and hair
naturally at only a fraction of the cost of mass-produced
preparations. And now is the time to discover it.

- Using fruit, herbs, flowers and vegetables grown at home,
bought or gathered from the wild, and ingredients from
your fridge or kitchen cupboard you will learn how easy
and fun it is to make a delightful range of original
beauty preparations including:

- **face creams** • **moisturising milks**
- **cleansing scrubs** • **skin tonics**
- **face packs** • **suntanning preparations**
- **lip salves** • **hair shampoos, conditioners and rinses**
- **hand and nail creams** • **bath oils**
- **colognes and floral waters**

0 7225 2498 6   £7.99

THE NATURAL FACE BOOK

Juliette Kando

If you are worried about losing your looks, there is now no need to resort to expensive, painful and risky cosmetic surgery. Follow this revolutionary facial workout plan and you can look years younger in just ten minutes a day!

Juliette Kando, a former ballet dancer, has developed a remarkable face and body balancing system which combines the principles of massage, acupressure, isometrics, calisthenics and yoga with herbalism and aromatherapy.

It can wipe years from your face in as little as two weeks.

THE NATURAL FACE BOOK

will show you step by step just how easy it is to:

- *Banish wrinkles, worry lines and angry frowns*
  - *revitalize drooping cheeks*
- *get rid of bags under the eyes and crows' feet*
  - *eradicate unsightly double chins*

More than just a natural facelift, Kando's holistic approach gives valuable hints on posture, sleep and self-image. You will not only look younger, you will see, hear, taste and think more clearly into the bargain.

Remember it is never too late to save your face – and change your life!

0 7225 2448 X   £7.99

The Book of Stress Survival

How to relax and live positively

Alix Kirsta

The Book of Stress Survival is the most useful and comprehensive reference available on stress management. Not only does it examine the causes and effects of stress it also shows how to pinpoint and reduce the stress in your life. With beautiful illustrations and clear step-by-step instructions, *The Book of Stress Survival* takes you through meditation and relaxation exercises to yoga and massage — essential skills for developing a stress-free lifestyle.+

- **Relax your body and your mind**
- **Release your positive energies**
- **Stress-proof your environment**
- **Plan a stress-free diet**
- **Develop confidence at work**
- **Improve your communication skills**
- **Experience peace of mind**
- **Overcome fear and anxiety**
- **Find time for yourself**
- **Feel loved and valued**

0 7225 2592 3   £8.99

Body Know-How

Jonathan Drake

At last a thoroughly practical, well-illustrated and effective guide to understanding and applying THE ALEXANDER TECHNIQUE in everyday activities.

Body Know-How explains how you can improve your physical and psycho-physical well-being through changing how you react to the stresses of daily life. You will also find out how you can recover efficient and proper use of your body, and so minimize pain, strain and injury.

Using THE ALEXANDER TECHNIQUE can help combat and prevent:

- **back and neck strain**
- **arthritis**
- **undue stress and fatigue**
- **headaches**
- **breathing difficulties**
- **hypertension**
- **gastro-intestinal problems**
- **many other psychosomatic disorders**

THE ALEXANDER TECHNIQUE teaches poise and confidence, which go hand in hand with co-ordination, and it is also of great value in learning and mastering skills.

0 7225 2394 7   £7.99